Green Computing and Predictive Analytics for Healthcare

Green Computing and Predictive Analytics for Healthcare

Edited by

Sourav Banerjee, Chinmay Chakraborty and Kousik Dasgupta

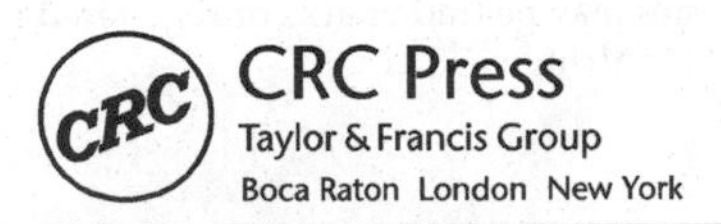

CRC Press is an imprint of the
Taylor & Francis Group, an **informa** business
A CHAPMAN & HALL BOOK

First edition published 2021
by CRC Press
6000 Broken Sound Parkway NW, Suite 300, Boca Raton, FL 33487-2742

and by CRC Press
2 Park Square, Milton Park, Abingdon, Oxon, OX14 4RN

CRC Press is an imprint of Taylor & Francis Group, LLC

ISBN: 978-0-367-32200-7 (hbk)
ISBN: 978-0-429-31722-4 (ebk)

Typeset in Palatino
by Deanta Global Publishing Services, Chennai, India

Contents

Preface

The main objective of this book is to explore the concepts of Green Computing, Big Data and the Internet of Things, along with recent research developments in the domain of healthcare. It also includes various applications and case studies in the field of computer science with the modern tools and technologies used. Population growth is a major challenge in maintaining and monitoring the different aspects of quality of service in healthcare. The efficient usage of these limited resources with moderate energy consumption has become more important. The major healthcare nodes are gradually becoming Internet of Things-enabled, and sensors, work data and the involvement of networking are creating smart campuses and smart houses. The book will cover chapters on the Internet of Things and Big Data technologies.

Chapter 1 discusses biomedical data monitoring under the Internet of Things, and also defines the health information sharing system whereby users not only can maintain and import their personal health records, but also can collate useful health web resources that are related to their personal diseases. This chapter deals with patients' record monitoring and smart healthcare data- sharing. Some issues must be considered in order to use cloud computing to quickly integrate medical big data into a database for easy analyzing, searching and filtering to obtain valuable information.

Chapter 2 highlights a new era of research that has been introduced where environment data sensing can be formulated and analyzed by technology and predict data output with a high probability of accuracy. Internet of Things is gradually being established as the new computing paradigm, which is bound to change our everyday working and living. This chapter focuses on the Internet of Things applications in healthcare management systems and also discusses the basic infrastructure requirements. The idea here is to develop a remote healthcare monitoring/advice system that can obtain data sets like body temperature, pulse rate, movement in the human body or some emergency blood pressure changes.

Chapter 3 introduces big data analytics and clustering methods for patients' data management. The different methodologies for big data and predictive analytics are explained. K-means, a traditional clustering algorithm, is applied for Electronic Health Records (EHRs) and discussed. A comparison of the various machine learning techniques for predicting diseases using the EHRs' dataset is included. Different issues with Electronic Health Records, such as interoperability, standardization, cost, security, privacy and confidentiality and processing abilities are also examined.

Chapter 4 proposes machine learning-based sudden cardiac death (SCD) prediction using statistical features. A literature survey suggests a growing interest among the research fraternity in detecting SCD. However, researchers are facing a challenge in resolving the solutions to predict SCD at an early stage. This work is aimed at early detection of sudden cardiac death symptoms. The proposed method is implemented in MATLAB and PYTHON software and validated with data from the MIT-BIH database to detect SCD.

Chapter 5 proposes robust segmentation methods for brain tissue segmentation. In this chapter, image segmentation is carried out with the use of fuzzy clustering and its variants' methods for classifying the three regions of the brain as grey matter, white matter and cerebrospinal fluid. Once the tissues are segmented, a similar diagnosis is useful for examining the presence of disorders in the brain. Brain image classification into tissues helps diagnose various illnesses such as tumor, stroke, multiple sclerosis and Alzheimer's disease. The machine learning techniques play a prominent position in the discipline of healthcare for producing data for various applications from the image input and classifying them in order to facilitate a positive diagnosis. Deep learning and Convolutional Neural Network, one of the machine learning approaches used, extracts the image facets for performing any kind of computer vision task, mainly medical applications, such as brain tissue classification for further prognosis and treatment.

Chapter 6 studies the energy-efficient and green Internet of Things for healthcare applications. Especially for the elderly, who have to consume multiple sets of medication every day, it becomes difficult to remember which to take and at what time. Monitoring elderly people for each and every second is a major issue that motivated us to investigate providing general solutions for healthcare systems using the Internet of Things. Due to the drastic increase in traffic and populations with limited resources, new technologies like the Internet of Things can be very useful in the field of healthcare monitoring and can also be used to make decisions before any critical event occurs. This study focuses on the basic and emerging technology of the Internet of Things, and various energy consumption techniques for Wireless Body Area Networks to enable the use of the green Internet of Things for various applications.

Chapter 7 explains e-health security in terms of the Internet of Things system and blockchain technology. The authors have also included various aspects like security engineering, cryptographical measures and cloud technology in the following sections. Interoperability, preservation of privacy and trust and authentication are the approaches used for maintaining the security of the e-health system against vulnerabilities and various attacks.

Chapter 8 discusses the domestic medical tourism system under the modern healthcare system in India. The author studies the documented features of the medical tourism sector in the state and analyzes its possible implications for domestic healthcare in Jaipur, Rajasthan. A joint committee with proper representation for all the sectors, including the public health sector, could be beneficial for the improvement of medical tourism in the state.

Chapter 9 introduces edge computing using machine learning techniques in the Internet of Things. In this chapter, a thorough overview of using advanced machine learning approaches, namely Deep Learning, is used in the edge analysis domain for real-time data streams. Here several applications in the healthcare and industrial areas in the Internet of Things domain are illustrated briefly.

We are sincerely thankful to the Almighty for supporting and standing at all times with us, whether in good or tough times, and giving the means of accepting us. Starting from the call for chapters till the finalization of chapters, all the editors gave their contributions amicably, which was itself a positive sign of significant teamwork. The editors are sincerely thankful to all the members of CRC Press, especially Gagandeep Singh, Aastha Sharma and Sikha Garg for providing constructive input and allowing the opportunity to edit this important book. We are equally thankful to the reviewers, who hail from different places around the globe, who shared their support and stand firm on quality chapter submissions. The rate of acceptance we have kept as low as was required to ensure the quality of work submitted by the author. The aim of this book is to support computational studies at the research and post-graduate level with open problem-solving techniques. We are confident that it will bridge the gap for them by supporting novel solutions to support in their problem-solving. In the end, the editors have taken the utmost care while finalizing the chapter to the book, but we are open to receive your constructive feedback, which will enable us to make any necessary changes in our forthcoming books.

About the Editors

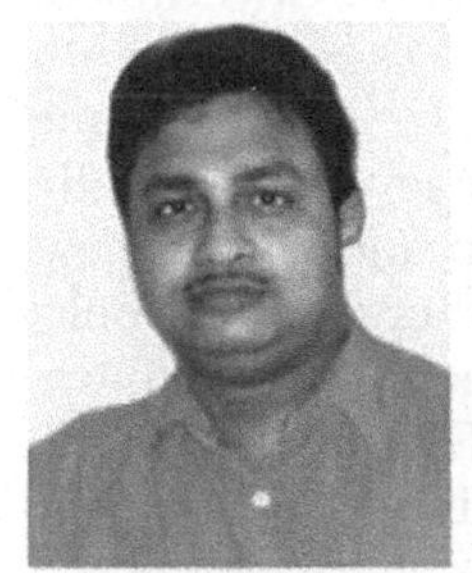

Sourav Banerjee achieved a PhD degree in Computer Science and Engineering from the University of Kalyani in 2017. He completed his BE in Computer Science and Engineering in the year 2004 and his MTech in Computer Science and Engineering in 2006. He is currently an Assistant Professor at the Department of Computer Science and Engineering of Kalyani Government Engineering College at Kalyani, West Bengal, India. He has authored numerous reputed unpaid SCI journal articles and book chapters and presented at international conferences. He has edited a book on Green Cloud Computing. His research interests include Big Data, Blockchain, Cloud Computing, Green Cloud Computing, Cloud Robotics, Distributed Computing and Mobile Communications and IoT. He is a member of IEEE, ACM, IAE and MIR Labs as well. He is an editorial board member of *Wireless Communication Technology*. He is the reviewer of *IEEE Transactions on Cloud Computing, Wireless Personal Communications, Journal of Ambient Intelligence and Humanized Computing, Journal of Computer Science, Journal of Supercomputing, Future Internet, International Journal of Computers and Applications, Personal and Ubiquitous Computing, Innovations in Systems and Software Engineering* and a lot of international conferences. He is connected with various international events, like the Workshop on Security and Privacy in Distributed Ledger Technology (IEEE SP-DLT). A number of international research scholars are supervised by him.

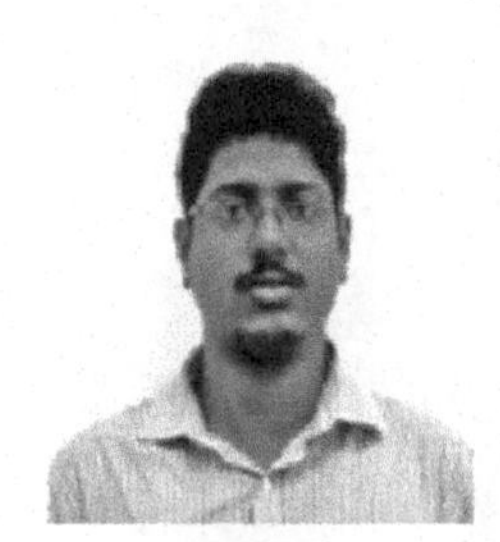

Chinmay Chakraborty is a Senior Assistant Professor in the Department of Electronics and Communication Engineering, BIT Mesra. His primary areas of research include Wireless Body Area Network, Internet of Medical Things, Energy-Efficient Wireless Communications and Networking, Point-of-Care Diagnosis. Prior to BIT, he worked at the Faculty of Science and Technology, ICFAI University, Agartala, Tripura, India as a senior lecturer. He worked as a Research Consultant in the Coal India project at Industrial Engineering & Management, IIT Kharagpur. He worked as a project coordinator of Telecom Convergence Switch project under the Indo-US joint initiative. He also worked as a Network Engineer in System Administration at MISPL under Global Teleservice Ltd, India. He received his PhD in Electronics & Communication from BIT Mesra, and his Master's from G.S. Sanyal School of Telecommunication, IIT Kharagpur. He authored the books *PSTN-IP Telephony Gateway for Ensuring QoS in Heterogeneous Networks* (2014), *Advanced Classification Techniques for Healthcare Analysis* (2019) and *Smart Medical Data Sensing and IoT Systems Design in Healthcare*. He is an Editorial Board Member for the *Journal of Wireless Communication Technology, Int. Journal of Telecomm. Engg.* etc. and also a member of the International Advisory Board for Malaysia Technical Scientist Congress and the Machine Intelligence Research Labs. He is a guest editor of the *Future Internet* journal special issue. He received the Outstanding Researcher Award from TESFA, 2016 and the Global Peer Review Award from Publons 2018 and also received the Young Faculty Award from VIFA 2018. He received the Young Research Excellence Award, Global Peer Review Award, Young Faculty Award and the Outstanding Researcher Award.

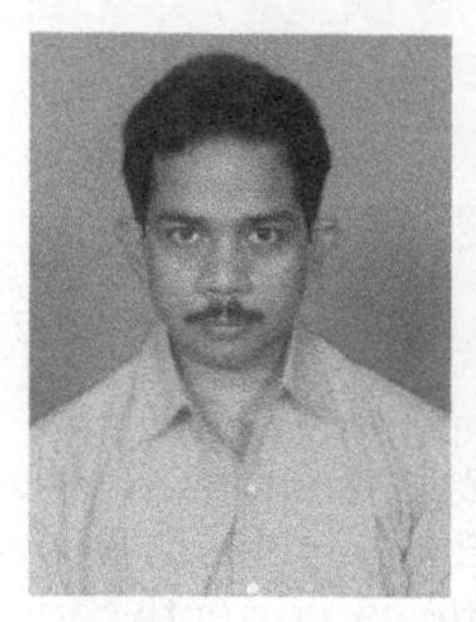

Kousik Dasgupta received his Bachelor of Engineering degree from Nagpur University, his Master's from West Bengal University of Technology and a Doctor of Philosophy in Engineering from the University of Kalyani. He has worked in industry for ABB, L&T, Lloyds Steel for three years in various capacities. Dr. Dasgupta is now Assistant Professor in the Department of CSE of Kalyani Government Engineering College. Apart from this, he has remained associated with the University of Kalyani, IIIT Kalyani, etc. as guest faculty from time to time. Dr. Dasgupta has been involved as the PI for several externally funded projects of AICTE and Technical Education and Department of Science and Technology, Government of West Bengal. He has co-authored three books and published about 28 papers in various journals and conference proceedings, both international and national. Dr. Dasgupta is a Life Fellow of the OSI, ISTE, ACM and IEEE, Computer Society, USA, and an Associate Member and Chartered Engineer [India] of the Institute of Engineers (India).

List of Contributors

B. Arthi
Associate Professor
SRM Institute of Science and Technology
Kattankulathur

M. Aruna
Assistant Professor
SRM Institute of Science and Technology
Kattankulathur

Prakash Banerjee
Department of Electrical and Electronics Engineering
University of Engineering and Management
Kolkata, India

Sourav Banerjee
Department of Computer Science and Engineering
Kalyani Government Engineering College
Kalyani, India

Sanjukta Bhattacharya
Department of Information Technology
Techno International Newtown
Kolkata, India

Chinmay Chakraborty
Department of Electronics and Communication Engineering
Birla Institute of Technology
Ranchi, India

Pramit Brata Chanda
Department of Computer Science and Engineering
Kalyani Government Engineering College
Kalyani, India

Surojit Das
Department of Computer Science
Kalyani College
Kalyani, India

S. Ananda Kumar
School of Computer Science and Engineering
Vellore Institute of Technology
Vellore, India

Subhankar Mishra
School of Computer Sciences
NISER and HBNI
Mumbai, India

Sudipta Paul
School of Computer Sciences
NISER and HBNI
Mumbai, India

Varsha Poddar
Department of Computer Science and Engineering
University of Engineering and Management
Kolkata, India

S. Srinivasa Rao
Department of Electronics and Communication Engineering
Malla Reddy College of Engineering and Technology
Hyderabad, India

V.S.K. Reddy
Department of Electronics and Communication Engineering
Malla Reddy College of Engineering and Technology
Hyderabad, India

Sukanya Roy
Department of Marketing
Indian School of Business
Mohali, India

R. Sandhiya
Department of Information Technology
Coimbatore Institute of Technology
Coimbatore, India

M. Sucharitha
Department of Electronics and Communication Engineering
Malla Reddy College of Engineering and Technology
Hyderabad, India

1

Healthcare Data Monitoring under Internet of Things

Chinmay Chakraborty and Sanjukta Bhattacharya

CONTENTS

1.1 Introduction

1.1.1 Healthcare Data – Efficient Storage of Big Data

In recent times, a large volume of data has been generated in various ways, which is why data overloading is a problematic issue and a suitable solution is needed to overcome this matter. Throughout the world, each and every day, an enormous amount of data is created, edited or updated and then consumed in several ways. Different organizations such as Google, International Data Corporation and Facebook have handled these data through various procedures for collection and storage purposes. Some giant companies store these data which include the browsing history, location of the user, bookmarks, current applications list, contacts, emails, etc. This large volume of data, which has the three characteristics variety, volume and velocity (known as the "3 Vs"), is defined as "Big Data" [1]. Here, "variety" indicates various unorganized and organized data such as video data, text data, transactional data, etc., whereas "velocity" defines how that much data are collected in a very small amount of time, meaning the data collection rate [2]. Throughout the whole world, the academic field and the industry are recently very much associated with generating and analyzing "Big Data" for several purposes. These massive amounts of data are not properly managed by traditional software, hardware or other platforms, because they exceed the previously used analytical and storage procedures. In recent times, several software programs and applications, which are technologically very advanced, fast and cost-effective, have been introduced to properly handle "Big Data" related to any critical computational task. These advanced applications include different types of modern techniques such as artificial intelligence (AI) and machine learning (ML), which are used to efficiently analyze the workable insights and also make proper decisions using "Big Data" [3]. These properly derived decisions are always used to give a more accurate impact in any field such as healthcare, transportation, privacy issues, etc., and to improve socio-economic life.

Healthcare is an area that is directly associated with human lives, where a small inaccuracy can be very much responsible for a large disaster for a human being. The healthcare industry is concerned with diagnosis, prevention and treatment procedures relating to human health. The healthcare industry depends on three major main components: health-related facilities, such as hospitals or clinics where the diagnosis and other treatments are delivered to the patients, medical experts, such as nurses or doctors or laboratory technicians, and financial firms. The medical experts or professionals are used to serve mainly four types of care, such as primary care where medical experts provide the first level of consultation to the patient, secondary care where highly skilled doctors are required for an acute level of care, tertiary care where advanced health-related investigations along with proper treatments are provided and quaternary care where exceptional and unusual disease diagnosis procedures followed by high-level surgical procedures take place [4]. At these four levels of care, health experts are responsible for generating large amounts of various kinds of medical data, such as the medical history of the patient, clinical data and personal data which is related to health issues. Nowadays, with the help of advanced techniques and applications, digitization is applicable in the storage and collection of all these medical data. In this case, the medical record, which is defined as an electronic health record (EHR), is efficiently used to store, capture, receive, retrieve, transmit and manipulate a patient's past, present or future mental and physical health data.

The healthcare segment is truly blessed through the usefulness of big data analytics, which not only efficiently manage vast amounts of medical data, but also help the medical industry in different ways, such as decreasing costs, preventing epidemics, etc. In the early days, data collection and gathering was really time-consuming and very costly, but nowadays managing this huge amount of data takes much less time with the help of different technological enhancements which are used to properly analyze patients' various health-related data, and also provide accurate information so that medical experts can take the right decision at a very early stage to prevent the disease, because prevention is always better than cure [5]. Using advanced technology, the cost of any long-term disease is also decreased in a very appreciable way.

1.2 Digitization of Healthcare-Oriented Big Data

The efficiency of different healthcare services, detection of medical errors, reduction in medical costs and quality of healthcare can be improved by using various healthcare data-related components, such as personal health records (PHR), electronic health records (EHR), medical practice management software, etc. Big data, along with its different advanced techniques, are able to acquire data from the web through some very intelligent and interesting methods. Basically, the EHR was introduced many years ago and in today's world, the value of EHR is constantly growing. It means that the healthcare industry, or, more accurately, the healthcare data, is very much dependent on different upcoming data management technologies. These varieties of advanced technology are also responsible for creating real-time health monitoring and biomedical systems through which medical data are sent to particular healthcare providers [6]. Massive amounts of data are generated by these sophisticated systems which are then properly analyzed and stored to correctly provide real-time healthcare. These highly specialized information technology-based systems, along with big data concepts, are used to improve medical costs and healthcare outcomes. In the case of biomedical research, different types of biological experiments and biological examinations are actually responsible for producing and storing medical data. The amount of this medical data is extremely large, which is very much essential to understanding any biological architecture or processes, such as two different technologies like genome-wide association studies and next-generation sequencing that are integrated with each other for the proper decoding of human genetics. The medical data which are basically generated from next-generation sequencing are used to provide a lot of useful information through which many medical-related activities are going to be made much easier through efficient methods, such as recoding or observation of biological-based events which are associated with critical diseases, fetching essential medical information from not only a single gene but also from the whole genome, rather than studying the transcription or expression of a single gene, it is better to study the expressions of all genes.

1.3 Healthcare – IoT and Mobile Health

Nowadays human life is flourishing, with various advanced and life-changing technologies such as the Internet of Things (IoT), big data, machine learning (ML), deep learning, etc. Most real-life areas are now habituated to these new technologies. IoT is one of the transformative technologies through which anything or anybody can be associated with or connected to each other anywhere and anytime. IoT is defined as a progressive technology where real-world smart objects are connected to achieve some capabilities, such as handling of storage and resources, proper organization of data and data-sharing in an effective way [7]. In the case of IoT, human beings or real-life material things such as sensors are connected to precisely achieve some specified tasks. Whenever this IoT-based connection is established, lots of data are generated that can be collected or interchanged for the proper use of real-life areas [8, 9]. Healthcare is one such segment that has developed enormously with the help of IoT in recent times.

Healthcare management in IoT is gaining popularity day by day. The integral part of IoT healthcare management is the sensors to capture the physiological parameters like body temperature, pulse rate, blood pressure, heartbeat, etc. [10]. These sensors are used as wearable IoT devices on human bodies to measure, capture and sometimes transmit health information from the human body in a wireless network environment. This transmitted information is generally stored and processed in a hub or smart gateways of the networks of body sensors called a body area network (BAN) or wireless body area network (WBAN) [11, 12]. These hubs or gateways use Raspberry Pi in current times to capture health information from these body sensors and send it to the health professionals located remotely far away from the patient for diagnosis. Also, the amount of data generated by the sensors could be enormous, so big data technology is applied to the local hubs or smart gateways or distant cloud servers, if included [13]. Cloud servers provide ongoing storage of the health information transmitted through the WBAN gateways or hubs. Health information which is not needed in real-time or emergency situations and could be used or analyzed in the future by health professionals for the purpose of treating the patient is usually stored in the cloud servers [14]. Emergency services or alerts which are time-sensitive are sometimes implemented through fog or edge computing devices situated and operated from an area very near to the WBAN rather than through the distant cloud [15]. These fog or edge computing devices serve as a local server to store time-sensitive data and act in real time to avoid the latency delay of the cloud in case of a critical situation.

Healthcare is a major issue of concern in a country as populated as India. The number of health professionals to attend all the patients, especially in rural areas, is nowhere near to adequate. Also setting up all the infrastructures for modern healthcare solutions in rural areas is almost impossible. One early solution thought of was telemedicine, but it was discarded later due to the problems of poor video reception quality and high infrastructural and maintenance cost in remote areas [10]. Almost all diseases can be prevented and diagnosed to a large extent if vital signs, like blood pressure, body temperature, pulse rate, respiration rate, blood oxygen saturation level, etc., are monitored regularly. The introduction of IoT in healthcare is proposed as a highly viable solution to this phenomenon. There are sensors invented that are wearable by the human body to capture the vital signs and transmit them to local servers connected through the wireless network, where the data can be stored, processed and monitored. These local servers are connected to remote machines through the internet and all or part of the information can be stored there so the health professionals connecting to these remote servers through the internet from anywhere at any time can check all the patients' information and diagnosis without checking the patient physically. This whole process of connecting sensor nodes, local devices where information from these nodes is processed and remote machines or servers are accessible to health professionals, is a revolution in healthcare. If this is implemented successfully, it will reduce the cost and quality of healthcare remarkably [10].

In the modern world, the whole universe is defined as the digital world and this world is connected through smart gadgets such as computers, mobiles, laptops, smartwatches, tablets, etc. Among all these gadgets, the popularity of mobiles is increasing tremendously day by day, and that is the reason that medical segments are also very dependent on mobile technology; this was formerly known as mobile health or "m-health" [16]. This mobile health has shown its ability to correctly identify several diseases including chronic diseases like cancer, diabetes, physical disorders, asthma, cystic fibrosis, Alzheimer's, etc. and can also help by providing high-end treatment facilities and innovative prevention procedures [17]. The patients, doctors and healthcare providers communicate through this mobile-based platform for managing the healthcare sector. Various giant organizations such as Google or Apple have been already developed innovative healthcare applications such as Google Fit or Apple's ResearchKit etc. These advanced applications are used for each and every aspect of any medical-related issues where patients, hospitals, medical professionals and healthcare providers are connected to each other for the betterment of the medical area, such as maintaining a healthy lifestyle, direct communication between patients and doctors for better clarification, etc.

IoT is playing a major role in the healthcare system via the internet and it operates in sensor networks, smartphone devices, wireless networking and cloud frameworks. IoT can also cover different areas like home, environment, cities, energy, retail, agriculture, logistics, industry and healthcare sectors also. An IoT system has intelligent interfaces that are permitted to send content and have a unique identifier (IP address/URI). In the field of healthcare, the IoT provides health and fitness monitoring and wearable electronics. The wearable IoT devices permit periodic non-invasive monitoring of the physiological parameters. The request-response is also used for healthcare data delivery. IoT systems consist of many components like device, controller service, resources, database, web service, stateless/stateful, bi-directional/uni-directional, request-response/full-duplex, TCP connection, scalability, header overhead and analysis. IoT devices can interchange data among the connected devices. The upper layer of IoT provides process-to-process communication using various protocols like hypertext transfer protocol, constrained application protocol, WebSocket, message queue telemetry transport, extensible messaging and presence protocol, data distribution service and advanced message queuing protocol. The visualization of IoT data is performed on cloud-based applications. With IoT systems having complex structures, the main requirements are enhanced reliability, many system configurations, statistical data monitoring, automating configuration, system-based configuration and data-retrieving configuration. The biomedical data can be processed from nodes to cloud frameworks, as shown in Figure 1.1.

The most enabling technologies of IoT are wireless sensor networks (WSN) and cloud computing. A WSN consists of nodes, router/gateway and coordinators. The cloud computing framework gives storage resources, computing and resources on an on-demand basis. Chen et al. [18] discussed real-time online vehicle diagnostics and early fault measurement method. Telehealth, telemedicine, e-health, m-health, digital medicine, precision medicine, digital health and personalized medicine are used effectively. The telemedicine tool plays an important role in chronic wound monitoring using the m-health scenario [19]. Health 4.0 technology is performing well and handles the critical medical infrastructure. The major principles of Health 4.0 are modularity, real-time capability, virtualization, service orientation, decentralization and interoperability. The mobile IoT manages asthma disease, heart disease and diabetes and processes medical data for monitoring. This data is associated with pharmaceutical and non-pharmaceutical therapy. The smart inhaler enhances the efficiency of therapy, minimizes serious incidents, increases quality healthcare, enhances documentation and reduces hospitalization. Asthma management needs sufficient adherence to therapy, monitoring of asthma control and prevention of environmental triggers [20]. Chakraborty et al. [21] discussed the telemedicine-based wireless body area network platforms for remote health monitoring. The various types of biomedical sensors have been presented. In digital healthcare systems, the patients demand accurate diagnosis. It depends on continuous patient monitoring. The patient's vital signs are taken by computerized devices and processed to the patient data management system (PDMS) server. The biomedical images are kept at the hospital's central node, i.e. picture archiving and communication system (PACS) in the form of DICOM (digital images and communication in medicine) files. This file is supported by multidimensional images and provides rich meta clinical information like demographic information, parameter acquisition, operator's

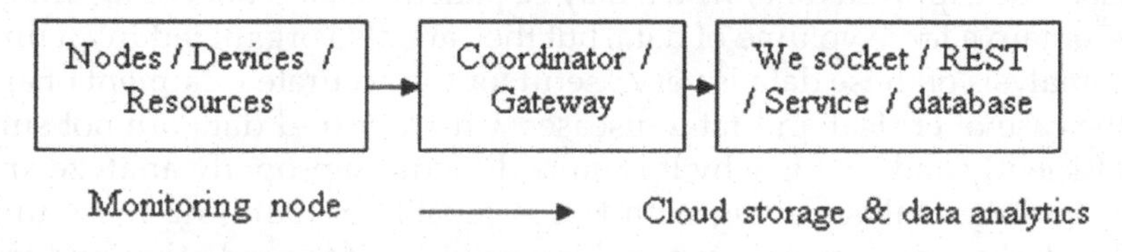

FIGURE 1.1
Route for data processing.

identifiers, practitioners, image dimensions [22]. M-health data is processed wirelessly to IoT servers for storage, transmitting and receiving. The smart sensed data management under IoT-healthcare is the most promising nowadays [23]. The main features of m-health are as follows: (a) compact and easy-to-wear (TICKR – heart rate monitor; Fitbit Surge, Forerunner 920XT – smartwatch; iBGStar – blood sugar meter); (b) IP-enabled and wireless connectivity (the Infrared Data Association, Nike+, Bluetooth Low Energy, ANT, ZigBee, near-field communication, Wi-Fi); and (c) low power consumption [24].

1.4 Management of Big Data

1.4.1 Electronic Medical Record (EMR) or Electronic Health Record (EHR)

Patient-related data such as socio-behavioral data, medical imaging data and environmental data can be collected in several ways in recent days. EHR is one of the efficient ways through which millions of files of medical data or patient-related data are collected and stored in an organized way. EHR has several characteristics which are very much related to healthcare areas. For example, the data which are collected and stored through EHR are very informative because these data, which may be prescriptions or any diagnosis report, actually contain various demographics, clinical reports, allergy results, etc. These informative medical data are very important to medical practitioners for identifying any critical diseases. Identifying any diseases at a very early stage can increase the chances of curing them, and the skills of medical experts can be improved day by day. Medical professionals are able to recognize any underlying diseases or genetic disorders through this informative data in the EHR, and then continuous monitoring or daily medical assistance may also be arranged to provide the patient with the best healthcare. Chances of errors are decreased, which are always blessings to human life, such as with accurate drug doses or proper vaccinations. Medical experts are sufficiently efficient with the help of the electronics platforms to focus on periodic checkups, to identify any ambiguity within the laboratory report or to recognize and start treatment for any deadly disease like cancer at the very beginning. Various healthcare and health insurance providers are introduced to patients for better treatment. Unauthorized activity related to healthcare is also reduced with the help of an EHR facility. EHR is used to increase the facility of paperless medical documents, decrease the total amount of time and, of course, reduce medical costs which is beneficial for everyone.

1.4.2 Healthcare Analytics

Analysis of medical data is truly essential for both the patients as well as medical professionals. Most of the captured data, which may be patient-related data or laboratory reports, do not only contain a large volume of data, but they are also organized in an unstructured way. Proper analysis of these data is very useful for the accurate treatment of any diseases mainly in the case of critical and fatal diseases. Unstructured data are not suitable to be dealt with efficiently and that is why it is quite difficult to properly analyze any unstructured data. Big data analysis along with ML is capable of handling these unstructured data and also derives correct decision-making solutions for prediction and treatment in the medical area.

In the case of big data, different formats and structure-based data are generated very quickly. The main challenge is to properly handle this large volume of data efficiently, because the healthcare or biomedical segments are very sensitive with regard to time and accuracy. These medical data must be captured in such a way that they are easily approachable and available to any scientific community. In big data applications, high-end, powerful hardware and software are always required for clinical-based setup. At the same time, many experts from different backgrounds such as information technology, mathematics, biology, statistics, etc. who have enough knowledge in their respective fields and are sufficiently experienced to properly deal with this advanced computing tool-based clinical setup are also essential. The huge amount of collected data is present and accessible in cloud-based storage with the help of some software tools which were previously installed in that storage and developed by analytically based tool developers. These tools are made of advanced ML and data-mining techniques which are truly useful for acquiring, storing, analyzing and visualizing the big data in such a way that it can easily and accurately integrate, annotate or arrange the complex data for much better decision-making and understanding purposes. Another challenge in the analysis of big data is the heterogeneous nature of data. The most suitable platforms to assist the analysis of big data are the clusters that are made of high computational power and accessed with the help of grid computing infrastructure. It is one of the reasons that cloud computing is one of the systems which is actively used in big data concept. Cloud computing has several characteristics, such as high reliability, autonomy, composability, scalability, etc. which are really useful for the big data area, because these platforms can do various roles at the same time e.g., they can receive data from different sensors, properly analyze and then interpret data and provide the appropriate person easy and understandable visualization. Advanced and efficient techniques based on AI and ML approaches are needed for the implementation and analysis of big data within the clusters. Fog computing and mobile edge computing cloudlets are some good technological platforms or tools for big data analysis. Lastly, a high-level programming language such as R, Python, etc. is required for the proper implementation of AI or ML-based algorithms. Professionals from trades like information technology and biology are required for big data-oriented platforms like Apache Spark or Hadoop.

1.5 Medical Data Analysis and Disease Predictions through ML

ML is one of the most powerful emerging technologies that has immense potential in every sector of everyday life, including the healthcare field. This technology consists of various techniques and applications which are not only used to solve many medical problems, but also to help accurately diagnose the diseases. In the case of the medical field, the chances of identifying the correct symptoms of the diseases are the most challenging issues. Due to the unavailability of medical data, such as insufficient data, missing data or unstructured data, the correct recognition of diseases is a most challenging job nowadays. These problems in identifying diseases are now much reduced with the help of ML, where the continuous learning process is very much effective for a proper understanding of medical data. ML is used to handle a huge amount of medical data very accurately in a minimum amount of time.

More challenges are associated with the ML-based medical imaging field and that is the reason that most of the researchers are dedicating their research toward this area. The biomedical or health informatics area consists of many fields such as medicine, biology, computational science, etc. The basic step of an ML-based pipeline structure is preprocessing, which consists of some techniques such as reduction, transformation, integration, etc. and these techniques are used to deal with medical data-related problems, such as inconsistent data, noisy data or missing data, etc. Modeling is defined as the next step of ML architecture which is responsible for building various data models like statistical models, probabilistic models, etc. where these models are used to efficiently fetch the patterns or features from the collected medical data. The next stage is known as evaluation, where the efficiency, complexity and technical correctness are checked. Next is the validation stage, and after that, the verification procedure is generated to examine the construction and working flow of the model. After that, medical coding is required, where the data are systematically classified into proper alphanumeric codes for accurate and efficient identification of medications, diagnosis, laboratory tests, procedures and additional clinical properties [25]. Nowadays the medical field is growing every day through the proper use of several techniques of ML which are genuinely introduced to improve and manage the medical sector. Using ML, public health is more protected due to proper detection, and after that, correct prevention, of any diseases or infectious outbreaks very quickly and accurately. Several gene sequencing methods have been invented to properly capture DNA sequences and perform any genome-oriented association for the investigations of the microbiome or any complex diseases. Any critical analysis or investigations from the historical and unstructured data can easily be done to correctly detect the patient's health, and at the same time, personalized care is also possible with the help of ML techniques. Health security issues are also taken advantage of whenever ML methods are applied to medical fields [26].

1.6 Applications of Big Data in the Medical Field

The production of Higgs bosons at the Large Hadron Collider can be performed now by generating huge amounts of collision data that needs to be filtered and analyzed, an example of quantum computing, a potential solution for big data analysis nowadays. The quantum annealing for ML, a successful quantum approach, helps to reduce human intervention and to increase the accuracy of assessing particle-collision data by the implementation of a combination of ML and quantum computing with a programmable quantum annealer. One of the quantum approaches that could find applications in many areas of science is new data classification, which is classified by the implementation of a quantum support vector for both acquiring skills and categorization stages [27]. Similarly, there are many applications of quantum approaches regarding healthcare e.g., implementation of a recurrent quantum neural network (RQNN) [28] to increase signal reparability in electroencephalogram (EEG) signals; execution of quantum annealing to intensity-modulated radiotherapy beamlet intensity optimization along with quantum sensors and quantum microscopes [29]. Three main applications of the big data concept are discussed below.

(1) Nowadays, big data is of huge assistance in healthcare to solve the proportion of staff and patients, which is a fundamental and traditional problem any shift manager often faces in hospital. A Forbes article specifies that four hospitals in Paris, part of the Assistance Publique – Hôpitaux de Paris have been applying

data from various sources to predict the expected number of patients daily and hourly in each hospital. Data scientists used "time series analysis" techniques for hospital admission records, cooperating with the researchers to get an up-to-date pattern of hospital admission rates so they could then apply "machine learning" to obtain the highly accurate algorithms that forecast the particular directions of future hospital admissions. In addition, from all this work, Forbes states:

> The result is a web browser-based interface designed to be used by doctors, nurses and hospital administration staff – untrained in data science – to forecast visit and admission rates for the next 15 days. Extra staff can be drafted in when high numbers of visitors are expected, leading to reduced waiting times for patients and better quality of care.

(2) Electronic Health Records (EHRs) are the most extensive application of big data analysis in medical science, sharing records of all kind of medical test results for every patient, digitally, in a one modified file, via secure information systems to providers from the private and public sector. With EHRs, doctors can easily implement any changes in any patient's medical record without paperwork and data repetition. EHRs can warn and remind about the next lab test of a patient and track prescriptions to observe how strictly a patient has been following the doctor's orders. The European Commission is focused on changing this by 2020, with an ambitious Directive. The practical scenario should become a Centralized European Health Record System. Kaiser Permanente could provide a model to follow for the EU, as they follow the lead of the US by implementing a system called "Health Connect" to make it easier to use EHRs and to share data widely. As per the McKinsey report on big data, healthcare states that "The integrated system has improved outcomes in cardiovascular disease and achieved an estimated $1 billion in savings from reduced office visits and lab tests".

(3) One of the crucial functions of Big Data Analysis in healthcare is "real-time alerting". Medical practitioners get analytical medical data and an advisory procedure for making prescriptive decisions, with the technical support of Clinical Decision Support software. Doctors do not welcome the system of patients staying in hospitals, because of expensive inpatient treatments. Analytics has the potential to proceed through a new method as one of the business intelligence buzzwords in 2020, by collecting patient's health data and sending that data to the cloud continuously. The data, which details the state of health of the general public, will be accessible in the database for doctors, to allow them to compare this data in a socio-economic context, and to modify updated delivery strategies. Organizations and healthcare managers will keep observing the database with their developed tools and will react to any unpleasant outcome. There are lots of practical examples, like if a patient's blood pressure increases unnaturally, the system will send a real-time alert to the doctors to take immediate action to control that patient's blood pressure. Another example is Asthmapolis, which has started to use inhalers with GPS-enabled trackers, to identify the trends of asthma in an individual and in the larger population. For the improvement of asthma treatment, data from the CDC is being used in conjunction with the data of Asthmapolis.

Apart from the above applications, there exist other frameworks or applications which are also useful and important in the medical field. Some of them are described here. One of the applications of big data analytics in the medical segment is the prevention of the misuse of opioids which cause many accidental and unnatural deaths. The other implementation is in personalized medical care for cancer patients, because constant caring and monitoring are very important for this type of chronic and critical disease. Cancer is a deadly disease that causes the deaths of thousands of people. Diabetes is defined as another deadly disease, and new applications have also been invented which are used to collect the contextual, behavioral and physiological data for evaluation purposes and to give the best care to the patients. Another application is strategic planning which is used to give more motivation to the patients so that the patients can cooperate with the treatment procedure and improve their lives. Next, the big data related framework is used to enhance the patient's engagement in different ways. In recent times, many patients are involved in checking their primary investigations by themselves using some smart techniques and gadgets which are truly useful to track and record some daily health-related symptoms, such as heart rate, blood pressure, weight, blood sugar, sleeping habits, etc. to accurately identify any chronic health risk. The next application is predictive analysis, where some smart tool is used to provide the patient's medical history, with full involvement of the patient, to the medical practitioners safely and securely so that they can efficiently predict the problem and also enhance the patient's health through their treatment process. The other applications are used to prohibit unnecessary and unauthorized access to medical data and also identify fraud cases with the help of advanced security. Applications are invented to correctly tackle and prevent arthritis problems, several important eye diseases, dengue outbreaks, etc. The next application is introduced to improve and enhance health-related laws in middle- and low-income countries. Applications have also been invented to properly manage and organize nutrition-based management. The next framework is implemented to tackle the clinics and hospitals properly, prevent human errors and reduce health costs as much as possible.

1.7 Analytics of Medical Data in the Mercantile Platform

Nowadays, different corporations and giant organizations are starting to implement big data along with ML and AI concepts for better analyzing purposes. Flatiron Health is one of the big corporations which has been serving as a medical analytics organization, mainly in cancer-related areas. Other giant organizations like Google Inc. and Oracle Corporation have started the development of platforms that are made from a distributed computing system and also cloud-oriented storage space [30]. Another big company, IBM, has also taken up the big data challenge and implemented it in delivering the ultimate accuracy level. IBM's Watson Health is a high-end AI-oriented platform through which medical data can be shared and then analyzed among researchers, hospitals and healthcare providers [31]. This platform uses the AI- and ML-oriented techniques to fetch maximum informative parts from minimum medical input and at the same time integrate some healthcare domain to easily get structured data. Pfizer along with IBM Watson have combined to develop a collaboration that is responsible to escalate the oncology-based discoveries and also deliver targeted drugs for cancer. In recent times, IBM Watson has also captured deep learning techniques along with AI, which are used to predict typical cancer-oriented genes and also interpret various critical genomic input data sets [32]. This AI-based platform has also shown its efficiency in the discovery of various drugs. In recent days, various companies, including small-cap, mid-cap or large-cap and the unlimited number of start-ups have started using the implementing strategy of big data and also providing more accurate solutions to healthcare fields. There are a variety of organizations defined as healthcare vendors who have begun to provide more commercial healthcare solutions. Linguamatics is a natural language processing (NLP)-oriented technique whose working strategy depends on an Interactive Text Mining Algorithm (I2E) which is responsible for fetching and then analyzing the information more quickly than any other tools; no specialized knowledge is required in this case. This particular approach is used to extract the necessary information from the unstructured data and also deliver a genetic relationship. When NLP is integrated with EHR, accurate and essential structured information is extracted from any unstructured medical data. AYASDI is also one such big medical vendor that has developed and then implemented an AI-oriented platform, along with a suitable application-based framework, with the help of ML technologies. This advanced vendor is used to provide many healthcare applications through which the analysis of healthcare is going to be made easier and the accuracy will be higher, such as managing and analyzing proper organization principles of different hospitals; managing clinically based variations, discussions between medical professionals and medical costs; analyzing high-risk decisions and treatments taken by medical experts, etc. At the same time, this healthcare vendor is used to deliver a combined application based on health population management and assessment. ML technology is the technological power behind this. AYASDI, which is used to accurately identify the risk-based drivers, predict the risks which will happen in the future and also provide the best solutions for any input of medical data.

1.8 Related Work

Khennoua et al. [33] discussed the correct adoption of different tools that are used for the analytical purpose of the EHR and also showed a survey of the implementation procedure of OpenEHR to properly investigate the adoption of healthcare analytics. Priyanka et al. [34] presented a thorough and detailed discussion on how the new advanced information-based concepts which are known as "big data" are used in the medical area to reduce medical costs, improve personalized medical care and refine the outcomes of the patient. Gai et al. [35] proposed an alert-based mechanism through the concept of big data, along with ontology which is used to help the medical practitioners to deliver an accurate diagnosis. The paper also discussed the proposed mechanism which is made of a new algorithm known as the Error Prevention Adjustment Algorithm (EPAA). Wu et al. [36] reported a review where EHR-based big data and omics characteristics, analytics procedures and challenges are mainly discussed, and at the same time also reviewed how big data are genuinely needed for precision-oriented medicine. Javier Andreu et al. [37] presented a complete overview of how big data, along with its powerful characteristics, are really a blessing, not only to the medical expert, but also to all the people who are directly or indirectly connected to healthcare. Asri et al. [38] described the influence of big data in the medical area through some pathways such as reduction of medical cost, enhancing the quality of medicine, improving the quality and values of healthcare, etc. This paper also discussed some healthcare solutions based on big data like Electronic Healthcare Predictive Analytics (e-HPA) and EHR, etc. Schatz [39] presented a review on population-based national health surveys which are used to show that big data analytics is very important for observing patients' health through some mobile applications. Goli et al. [40] proposed a model based on cloud computing and document-oriented databases which are used to store and then retrieve the big healthcare data more efficiently and accurately. Manogaran et al. [41] proposed an architecture that is used for storing the sensor-based data which are related to the human body and then properly processing the data for further medical applications. This proposed architecture is made of different technologies such as Apache HBase, Apache Flume and Apache Pig, while another technology, Apache Mahout, uses logistic regression-based Species Distribution Modeling algorithm (SGD) to build better diagnosis framework. Balamurugan et al. [42] discussed the different challenges associated with the Internet of Things (IoT) in the medical field and also showed various healthcare contributions of IoT. Viceconti et al. [43] discussed the five main problems associated with healthcare areas which are reduced or removed through the efficient integration of Virtual Physiological Human-based modeling and big data concepts. Zhang et al. [44] implemented a cyber-physical healthcare assistant system which is basically a patient-based medical application, as well as services known as Health-Cyber-Physical Systems (Health-CPS) based on big data and cloud computing. This Health-CPS consists of mainly three architectures: a unique layer which is used for data collection, and also the integration of customized medical services and public healthcare resources; a data-oriented and cloud-based platform for storing and then analyzing unstructured data; and a unified and unique Application Program Interface (API) for both the users and developers separately. Abouelmehdi et al. [45] reported a survey where the big data-related privacy and security issues in the healthcare domain are focused on, and at the same time, some new methods which are related encryption and data anonymization are also dealt with. Mancini [46] discussed the enormous potential and power of big data in medical areas, especially in the development of several drugs and personal medical care. Berger et al. [47] described a comparative and effective study on advanced big data analytics and its various future scopes which are very effective for the patients and the healthcare experts. Barrett et al. [48] presented a detailed description of exploring different big data-related applications and also presented two examples through which it can be shown how big data is used for the prevention of several diseases. Chen et al. [49] invented a model based on a convolutional neural network (CNN) with the help of a multimodal disease risk prediction (MDRP) algorithm which is known as the CNN-MDRP model. This model works with both unstructured and structured data medical data, and the disease prediction accuracy of this model reached 94.8% with great speed. Chouvarda et al. [50] discussed the main challenges of connected medical technologies which are mainly captured in chronic diseases. This connected ecosystem which is focused on healthcare has shown its benefits in several fields such as data feedback, analysis, integration, biosensors, database management, etc. Wyber et al. [51] reviewed the advantages and disadvantages of big data. At the same time, this paper also focused on how the use of big data in the medical ground effects in middle-income and low-income countries.

Hong et al. [52] demonstrated that how the PHR framework based on cloud computing and IoT platforms is truly effective for big data-oriented analysis purposes in the healthcare domain. Lv et al. [53] introduced two different mobile-based healthcare applications which are used to fetch data for use in Electronic Medical Records (EMR). One of the applications is efficient as a rehabilitation system for therapists, and the other one is effective for the improvement of patient-related care systems. Jalali et al. [54] evaluated how the Smarter Public Health Prevention System (SPHPS) based on Virtual Private Cloud (VPC) is implemented to properly address public health-related disparities. Peters et al. [55] described a detailed overview of EHR or EMR, including its advantages, disadvantages, development and future scope. Sokolova et al. [56] discussed the security and privacy issues of Personal Health Information (PHI), because PHI is associated with patient-related personal information. Sweet et al. [57] surveyed several issues of EHR and at the same time also focused on different constraints of meta-data in healthcare. Naqishbandi et al. [58] described how complex event processing, big data and IoT merge their power and potential to solve various complicated medical problems. Vuppalapati et al. [59] proposed a sensor-based integration system based on EHR and also presented a prototype-based solution along with some of the applications. West et al. [60] reviewed a new information-based visualization of EHR-based data, and compared the previous and new visualization techniques.

1.9 Challenges and Constraints Related to Healthcare-Based Big Data Concepts (Including Privacy and Security Issue)

There are several challenges, including the privacy and security issues that exist in big data when it is mainly used in the medical sector. Several methods and techniques are developed and used for the management and analysis purposes of big data, such as visualization-oriented solutions, real-time data streaming, data aggregation, etc. Some of the real-time big data-related constraints or challenges are discussed here. The first one is known as data-sharing, where mainly the patient-related data are the prime factor. It can be seen that the patients are often transferred from one clinic to another clinic due to some medical emergency, but the present clinic does not receive any previous medical data of the particular patient and that is why sometimes the diagnostic procedures do not meet with the patient's expectations. Some of the applications have already been developed such as Carequality, Fast Healthcare Interoperability Resource (FHIR), CommonWell, etc. which are used to share and access the medical data safely and easily. Still, there exist lots of medical data-related issues that can be reduced when a trustworthy, accurate and simple big data-oriented data exchange system is developed. The next constraint is the protection issue which is always a priority in healthcare. Medical data are very sensitive and that is why they must be secured from any unauthorized access. Various advanced security-based measures such as firewalls, multi-factor authentication, antivirus software, etc. are used nowadays for the protection of data. The next challenge is the data formatting issue. Each and every day, lots of medical data, clinical data and personal data are generated which are not only huge in amount, but also the structure and meaning of these data are not managed easily. For proper and accurate disease prediction purposes, it is essential to extract meaningful information from the collected data and organize the data in a structured format. Several advanced systems have been introduced as a solution to these data formatting problems, such as Current Procedural Terminology.

The next issue is the storage problem. Storing this huge amount of medical data is really a big challenge because most of the organizations and corporations prefer to store their data within their own storage. An IoT-based cloud storage platform is one of the most suitable solutions because this technology has been developed to provide reliability, safety, cost deduction, easier expansion and also disaster recovery. The next constraint is the image preprocessing which actually suffers from artifacts, noise and tampering. Medical imaging is also an extremely crucial weapon for the purposes of making a correct diagnosis and that is the reason that several methods are proposed and implemented to save medical images from any mishandling. The next one is that data must be scrubbed or cleansed to provide relevancy, accuracy, consistency, purity, correctness, etc. Most of the real-time acquired data do not satisfy these conditions and that is why various precise and sophisticated ML-based techniques are developed to fulfill these criteria. Data visualization is another constraint that is very useful in the case of medical data where histograms, charts and heat maps are widely acceptable. Generating meta-data is also important, especially when the big data are related to the medical area, because meta-data is used to easily generate some query and after that achieve their respective outcomes. The next challenge is accuracy, which is the most important matter in the healthcare area. Medical data are related to human health and a small inaccuracy in the prediction procedure can lead to a large disaster for a human life. Many frameworks and applications have been made to identify diseases with optimal accuracy.

1.10 Conclusion and Future Trends

This chapter discusses biomedical data monitoring using IoT frameworks. The different types of medical data can be processed from smart devices to cloud platforms. The data collection, generation and analysis are developed and improved in the medical field every day by using these improved technological systems. Big data is used to enhance patients' engagement in various ways. These ML-based techniques play an important role in healthcare because these techniques not only reduce medical costs, surprisingly, but also increase the accurate prediction of actual diseases. Various machine learning-based models are also developed for providing better diagnosis and treatment to the patients. Different smartphone applications are trying to give flexibility for medical information visualization and monitoring purposes. Secured medical data processing is the main challenge nowadays.

References

1. Amit B., Chinmay C., Anand K., and Debabrata B. 2019. Emerging trends in IoT and big data analytics for biomedical and health care technologies. *Handbook of Data Science Approaches for Biomedical Engineering*, Ch. 5., 121–152, Elsevier.
2. De M., Andrea, Marco G., and Michele G. 2016. A formal definition of Big Data based on its essential features. *Library Review*, 65, no. 3, 122–135.
3. Gubbi J., Rajkumar B., Slaven M., and Marimuthu P. 2013. Internet of Things (IoT): A vision, architectural elements, and future directions. *Future Generation Computer Systems* 29, no. 7, 1645–1660.
4. Gillum R.F. 2013. From papyrus to the electronic tablet: A brief history of the clinical medical record with lessons for the digital age. *American Journal of Medicine* 126, no. 10, 853–857.
5. Reisman M. 2017. EHRs: The challenge of making electronic data usable and interoperable. *Pharmacy and Therapeutics* 42, no. 9, 572.
6. Shameer K., Marcus A.B., Riccardo M., Benjamin S., Glicksberg J.W., Morgan, and Joel T.D. 2017. Translational bioinformatics in the era of real-time biomedical, health care and wellness data streams. *Briefings in Bioinformatics* 18, no. 1, 105–124.

7. Chakraborty C. 2019. Mobile Health (m-Health) for Tele-wound Monitoring, Anastasius M., Mobile Health Applications for Quality Healthcare Delivery, Ch. 5, 98–116, IGI Global A.
8. Poyen E.F.B., Amit K.B., B. Durga M., Imran A., Arghya S., and Awanish P.R. 2016. Density based traffic control. *International Journal of Advanced Engineering, Management Science* 2, no. 8, 1379–1384, Infogain Publication.
9. Crainic T. Gabriel M.G., and Jean Y.P. 2009. Intelligent freight-transportation systems: Assessment and the contribution of operations research. *Transportation Research Part C: Emerging Technologies* 17, no. 6, 541–557.
10. Garbhapu V.V., and Sundararaman G. 2017. IoT based low cost single sensor node remote health monitoring system. *Procedia Computer Science* 113, 408–415.
11. Maity S., Debayan D., and Shreyas S. 2017. Wearable health monitoring using capacitive voltage-mode human body communication. In *2017* 39th Annual International Conference of the IEEE Engineering in Medicine and Biology Society (EMBC), pp. 1–4. IEEE.
12. Yang G., Li X., Matti M., Xiaolin Z., Zhibo P., Li D.X., Sharon K.W., Qiang C., and Li R.Z. 2014. A health-IoT platform based on the integration of intelligent packaging, unobtrusive bio-sensor, and intelligent medicine box. *IEEE Transactions on Industrial Informatics* 10, no. 4, 2180–2191.
13. Manogaran G., Ramachandran V., Daphne L., Priyan M.K., Revathi S., and Chandu T. 2018. A new architecture of Internet of Things and big data ecosystem for secured smart healthcare monitoring and alerting system. *Future Generation Computer Systems* 82, 375–387.
14. Firouzi F., Amir M.R., Kunal M., Mustafa B., Geoff V.M., Wong P., and Bahar F. 2018. Internet-of-Things and big data for smarter healthcare: From device to architecture, applications and analytics, *Future Generation Computer Systems*, 78, no. 2, 583–586, Elsevier.
15. Rathore M.M., Awais A., Anand P., Jiafu W., and Daqiang Z. 2016. Real-time medical emergency response system: Exploiting IoT and big data for public health. *Journal of Medical Systems* 40, no. 12, 283.
16. Moore, Samuel K. 2001. Unhooking medicine [wireless networking]. *IEEE Spectrum* 38, no. 1, 107–108.
17. Nasi G., Maria C., and Claudia G. 2015. The role of mobile technologies in health care processes: The case of cancer supportive care. *Journal of Medical Internet Research* 17, no. 2, e26.
18. Chen S.H., Jhing F.W., YuRu W., John S., and Shao Y.K. 2011. The implementation of real-time on-line vehicle diagnostics and early fault estimation system. In *2011* Fifth International Conference on Genetic and Evolutionary Computing, pp. 13–16. IEEE.
19. Chakraborty C., Gupta B., and Ghosh S.K. 2016. Mobile telemedicine systems for remote patient's chronic wound monitoring. In *IGI Global: M-Health Innovations for Patient-Centered Care*, Ch. 11, pp. 217–243.
20. Boulet L.P., Daniel V., Yves M., and Juliet M.F. 2012. Adherence: The goal to control asthma. *Clinics in Chest Medicine* 33, no. 3, 405–417.
21. Chakraborty C., Bharat G., and Soumya K.G. 2013. A review on telemedicine-based WBAN framework for patient monitoring. *Telemedicine and e-Health* 19, no. 8, 619–626.
22. Mildenberger P., Eichelberg M., and Martin E. 2002. Introduction to the DICOM standard. *European Radiology* 12, no. 4, 920–927.
23. Chinmay C. 2019. Smart medical data sensing and IoT systems design in healthcare, *IGI Global Book Series—Advances in Healthcare Information Systems and Administration (AHISA)*, 1–288. doi: 10.4018/978-1-7998-0261-7
24. Almotiri S.H., Murtaza A.K., and Mohammed A.A. 2016. Mobile health (m-health) system in the context of IoT. In *2016* IEEE 4th International Conference on Future Internet of Things and Cloud Workshops (FiCloudW), pp. 39–42. IEEE.
25. Feldman K., Louis F., Xian W., Chao H., and Nitesh V.C. 2017. Beyond volume: The impact of complex healthcare data on the machine learning pipeline. Andreas H, Randy G., Massimo F., Vasile P., In *Towards Integrative Machine Learning and Knowledge Extraction*, pp. 150–169. Springer.
26. Clifton D.A., Niehaus K.E., Charlton P., and Colopy G.W. 2015. Health informatics via machine learning for the clinical management of patients. *Yearbook of Medical Informatics* 24, no. 01, 38–43.

27. Rebentrost P., Masoud M., and Seth L. 2014. Quantum support vector machine for big data classification. *Physical Review Letters* 113, no. 13, 130503.
28. Gandhi V., Girijesh P., Damien C., Laxmidhar B., and Thomas M.G. 2013. Quantum neural network-based EEG filtering for a brain–computer interface. *IEEE Transactions on Neural Networks and Learning Systems* 25, no. 2, 278–288.
29. Reardon S. 2017. Quantum microscope offers MRI for molecules. *Nature News* 543, no. 7644, 162.
30. Valikodath N.G., Paula A.N.C., Paul P., Lee D.C. Musch L.M.N., and Maria A.W. 2017. Agreement of ocular symptom reporting between patient-reported outcomes and medical records. *JAMA Ophthalmology* 135, no. 3, 225–231.
31. Beckles G., David F.W., Arleen F.B., Edward W., Gregg A.J., Karter C., Kim R., Adams D., Monika M., Safford, Mark R.S., and Theodore J.T. 2007. Agreement between self-reports and medical records was only fair in a cross-sectional study of performance of annual eye examinations among adults with diabetes in managed care. *Medical Care*, 45, no. 9, 876–883.
32. Echaiz J.F., Candice C., Jeffrey P.H., Hilary M.B., and Jonas M. 2015. Low correlation between self-report and medical record documentation of urinary tract infection symptoms. *American Journal of Infection Control* 43, no. 9, 983–986.
33. Khennou F., Youness I.K., and Nour E.H.C. 2018. Improving the use of big data analytics within electronic health records: A case study based openEHR. *Procedia Computer Science* 127, 60–68.
34. Priyanka K., and Nagarathna K. 2014. A survey on big data analytics in health care. *International Journal of Computer Science and Information Technologies* 5, no. 4, 5865–5868.
35. Gai K., Meikang Q., Li C.C., and Meiqin L. 2015. Electronic health record error prevention approach using ontology in big data. In *2015 IEEE 17th International Conference on High Performance Computing and Communications*, pp. 752–757. IEEE.
36. Wu P.Y., Chih W.C., Chanchala D.K., Janani V., Ryan H., and May D. W. 2017. Omic and electronic health record big data analytics for precision medicine. IEEE. *IEEE Transactions on Biomedical Engineering* 64, no. 2, 263–273.
37. Andreu P., Javier C.C.Y.P., Robert D.M., Stephen T.C.W., and Guang Z.Y. 2015. Big data for health. *IEEE Journal of Biomedical and Health Informatics* 19, no. 4, 1193–1208.
38. Asri H., Hajar M., Hassan A.M., and Thomas N. 2015. Big data in healthcare: Challenges and opportunities. In *2015* International Conference on Cloud Technologies and Applications (CloudTech), pp. 1–7. IEEE.
39. Schatz B. 2015. National surveys of population health: Big data analytics for mobile health monitors. *Big Data* 3, no. 4, 219–229.
40. Goli M.Z., Morteza S.J., and Mohammad K.A. 2016. An effective model for store and retrieve big health data in cloud computing. *Computer Methods and Programs in Biomedicine* 132, 75–82.
41. Manogaran G., and Daphne L. 2018. Health data analytics using scalable logistic regression with stochastic gradient descent. *International Journal of Advanced Intelligence Paradigms* 10, no. 1–2, 118–132.
42. Balamurugan S., Madhukanth R., Prabhakaran V.M., and Gokul K.R.S. 2016. Internet of health: Applying IoT and big data to manage healthcare systems. *International Research Journal of Engineering and Technology* 310, 732–735.
43. Viceconti M., Peter H., and Rod H. 2015. Big data, big knowledge: Big data for personalized healthcare. *IEEE Journal of Biomedical and Health Informatics* 19, no. 4, 1209–1215.
44. Zhang Y., Meikang Q., Chun W.T., Mohammad M.H., and Atif A. 2015. Health-CPS: Healthcare cyber-physical system assisted by cloud and big data. *IEEE Systems Journal* 11, no. 1, 88–95.
45. Abouelmehdi K., Abderrahim B.H., and Hayat K. 2017. Big healthcare data: Preserving security and privacy. *Journal of Big Data* 5, no. 1, 1–18.
46. Mancini M. 2014. Exploiting big data for improving healthcare services. *Journal of e-Learning and Knowledge Society* 10, no. 2, 23–33.
47. Berger M.L., and Vitalii D. 2014. Big data, advanced analytics and the future of comparative effectiveness research. *Journal of Comparative Effectiveness Research* 3, no. 2, 167–176.
48. Barrett M.A., Olivier H., Robert A.H., and Nancy E.A. 2013. Big data and disease prevention: From quantified self to quantified communities. *Big Data* 1, no. 3, 168–175.

49. Chen M., Yixue H., Kai H., Lu W., and Lin W. 2017. Disease prediction by machine learning over big data from healthcare communities. *IEEE Access* 5, 8869–8879.
50. Chouvarda I.G., Dimitrios G.G., Irene L., and Nicos M. 2015. Connected health and integrated care: Toward new models for chronic disease management. *Maturitas* 82, no. 1, 22–27.
51. Wyber R., Samuel V., William P., Priya M., Temitope F., and Leo A.C. 2015. Big data in global health: Improving health in low-and middle-income countries. *Bulletin of the World Health Organization* 93, 203–208.
52. Hong J., Peter M., and Jonghwa S. 2017. Interconnected personal health record ecosystem using IoT cloud platform and HL7 FHIR. In *2017* IEEE International Conference on Healthcare Informatics (ICHI), pp. 362–367. IEEE.
53. Lv Z., Javier C., and Pablo G. 2016. Bigdata oriented multimedia mobile health applications. *Journal of Medical Systems* 40, no. 5, 120.
54. Jalali A., Olusegun A.O., and Christopher M.B. 2012. Leveraging cloud computing to address public health disparities: An analysis of the SPHPS. *Online Journal of Public Health Informatics* 4, no. 3, 1–7.
55. Peters S.G., and Munawwar A.K. 2014. Electronic health records: Current and future use. *Journal of Comparative Effectiveness Research* 3, no. 5, 515–522.
56. Sokolova M., and Stan M. 2016. Personal privacy protection in time of big data. Matwin S., Mielniczuk, In *Challenges in Computational Statistics and Data Mining*, pp. 365–380. Springer.
57. Sweet L.E., and Heather L.M. 2013. Electronic health records data and metadata: Challenges for big data in the United States. *Big Data* 1, no. 4, 245–251.
58. Naqishbandi T.C., Imthyaz S., and Qazi S. 2015. Big data, CEP and IoT: Redefining holistic healthcare information systems and analytics. *International Journal of Engineering Research and Technology* 4, no. 1, 1–6.
59. Vuppalapati C., Anitha I., and Santosh K. 2016. The role of big data in creating sense EHR, an integrated approach to create next generation mobile sensor and wearable data driven electronic health record (EHR). In *2016 IEEE Second International Conference on Big Data Computing Service and Applications (BigDataService)*, pp. 293–296, IEEE.
60. West V.L., David B., and Hammond W.E. 2015. Innovative information visualization of electronic health record data: A systematic review. *Journal of the American Medical Informatics Association JAMIA* 22, no. 2, 330–339.

2

A Framework for Emergency Remote Care and Monitoring Using Internet of Things

Varsha Poddar

CONTENTS

2.1 Introduction

Internet of Things (IoT) is an environment of connected physical objects accessible through an internet connection. The "thing" in IoT can be a person, a sensor or a connected electronic device (with built-in sensor) that can be accessed through a central access point or a common connected device [1]. The wearables (sensors) would be able to sense data, transfer data or process the collected data set. The embedded technology will help the devices to interact with their internal states and with their external environment, which in turn is used for decision-making based on some logical input from a data set. When these devices represent themselves digitally, they can be controlled or monitored from anywhere, and using that property of embedded devices, decision-making in a suitable environment is established or centralized as a system-specific controller. The connectivity then helps us capture more data from distant and remote places, thus ensuring more ways of increasing efficiency and improving safety and IoT security. IoT can help organizations reduce costs through improved process efficiency, asset utilization and productivity. With improved tracking of devices using sensors and connectivity, they can benefit from real-time insights and analytics, which help them in making smarter decisions digitally [2]. The growth and convergence of data, processes and things on the internet will make such connections more relevant and important, creating more opportunities for people, business and industries. IoT enables companies to reduce labor costs and automate processes. It also cuts down on waste and improves service delivery, making it less expensive to manufacture and deliver goods as well as offering transparency for customer transactions.

IoT in the present scenario touches every aspect of life, including healthcare, finance, retail and manufacturing [2]. Likewise, smart cities help in reducing waste and improving customized accuracy in decision-making. In the broader concept, an IoT system does its job in three steps: collect data; collate data and transfer them; and finally, analyze data to take respective actions.

The benefits of using IoT can be summarized as monitoring the overall business process and improving the customer experience with the system. It improves total employee productivity and saves money as well as time, while simultaneously making better decisions and generating more revenue. IoT encourages companies to rethink the ways they approach their businesses, industries and markets and gives them the tools to improve their business strategies [3]. IoT gives the ability to access information from anywhere, at any time, on or from any device and thus improves communication between connected electronic devices. Transferring data packets over the network saves time and money, and at the same time automating the task helps improve business quality services and reduces human intervention in the process. Similarly the use of IoT can bring in a few troubles when the number of connected devices increases and more information is shared between devices. The potential that a hacker could steal confidential information also increases [4]. Again, if there is a virus in the system, it's more likely that the connected devices will get corrupted. Since there's no international standard of compatibility for IoT, it is difficult for devices from different manufacturers to communicate with each other.

While IoT is considered to be one of the most promising and accurate data analysis and prediction real-time systems, the technology suffers from various security-based attacks and system issues. The technology offers a huge added value to the home automation, energy conservation, transportation and health sectors [5]. But there remain some threats on the systems while communicating or during data transfer. One interconnection is referred to as Healthcare IoT (H-IoT), where real-time monitoring is done to gather information based on which predictions are made or assistance is to offered for patients. For securing the things connected on the internet, generally machine learning (ML) algorithms are applied in different fields where the stages involve identifying security vulnerabilities, identifying patterns in order to make predictions and identifying outliers [6].

In this chapter, a framework for an emergency remote care and monitoring system using IoT is proposed, using IoT devices connected to a central server for analysis and feedback. Section 2.2 gives a general overview of IoT architecture, and Section 2.3 does a literature survey of the work done in this domain. The proposed overall system that records the different real-time parameters and also sends an email/SMS alert whenever those readings go beyond critical values is described in Section 2.4. Results are given in Section 2.5, with concluding remarks and the future direction in Section 2.6.

2.2 The IoT Architecture and Applications

IoT is not just internet-connected consumer devices, but is a technology that builds systems capable of autonomously sensing and responding to stimuli from the real world without human intervention. The Internet of Things (IoT), which was once positioned as a niche technology for start-ups, is today a go-to technology for enterprises who want to transform their future business. IoT has already altered the way both professionals work and ordinary people live. Generally, automation and prediction are done on IoT-based systems to help people who may not seek prompt help for their environment or surroundings. To discuss its benefit to the users, IoT can be used in personal as well as business-oriented domains for customer services and experiences:

(i) Safety, control, efficiency
(ii) Better decision-making and predictions
(iii) Revenue generation, if run through business
(iv) Start with a small circle and increase the environment through connections

At the present time, to discuss healthcare issues, the patients have to visit health centers or advisors at regular intervals for checkups or diagnosis of specific symptoms or abnormalities. This can incur costlier services as people have to travel and select and be referred to specialists. From this, it has been clear that in availing of healthcare facilities, users need to invest a lot of their earnings into the area, and thereafter some confusion might also occur due to differences of opinion or the seriousness of the health issues monitored. If a system can be proposed where data input from wearable sensors could be used for predicting what is wrong, or whether there is any abnormality, then users can save both time and money invested in door-to-door diagnosis and prediction. The users can be accommodated from a remote location without an expert being present. Their location as well as their health issue can be tracked via an IoT-oriented approach, and predictive measures as well as analysis will be provided at regular time intervals. The various stages in an IoT environment for data acquisition and analysis are explained in this section. This stage details the working of the systems.

2.2.1 Stage 1 (Sensors/Actuators)

A "thing" in the context of IoT should be equipped with sensors and actuators, thus giving it the ability to emit, accept and process signals in order to collate the data sets for further decision-making and processing [7].

2.2.2 Stage 2 (Data Acquisition Systems)

The data from the sensors starts in an analog form, which needs to be aggregated and converted into digital streams for further processing. *Data acquisition systems* perform these data aggregation and conversion functions.

2.2.3 Stage 3 (Edge Analytics)

Once IoT data has been digitized and aggregated, it may require further processing before it enters the data center. This is where edge analytics comes in [8]. Edge analytics can be shaped as tools sitting in the sensor device or the acquisition device itself to process and fetch output there without sending it further to the cloud for analysis and decision-making. For example, a light sensor at a traffic light can be built with intelligent monitoring for traffic management. Devices are designed to contain their own analytical capabilities to this end.

2.2.4 Stage 4 (Cloud Analytics)

Data that needs more in-depth processing gets forwarded to physical data centers or cloud-based systems.

The proliferation of healthcare-specific IoT products opens up immense opportunities. The huge amount of data generated by these connected devices holds the potential to transform healthcare [9, 10]. Here, IoT has a four-step architecture basically used for acquiring and gathering information about healthcare aspects digitally and then analyzing them for logical decision-making. The stages include the data capturing stage, data aggregation, standardization and analyzing for making predictions [2]. IoT is redefining healthcare by ensuring better care, improved treatment outcomes and reduced costs for patients, and better processes and workflows, improved performance and patient experience for healthcare providers. The major benefits of IoT in healthcare include improved treatment, faster disease diagnosis, proactive treatment, drugs and environment management cost reduction and error reduction rate [11–13]. For remote patient monitoring, personal health data and medical data investigatory reports are collected from an individual in a remote location and are transmitted later to a service provider (hospitals) at a different location for related support. In this way the provider can track or maintain the healthcare data even after the patient is released after treatment [10]. Thus, the patient's data or care can be maintained by the service provider without making them go to their individual offices, etc. "mHealth" [14, 15] means the practice of patient monitoring or serving as supported by cell phones or PDAs. Smart health applications can range from targeted text messages to wide-scale alerts about disease outbreaks or other options that you choose for yourself. The integration of healthcare monitoring using an IoT-based system can be optimized as wearable or portable devices connect to the cloud, and pull and analyze the collected real-time data from patients remotely. This is to monitor vital health indicators collected by portable devices, charts and diagram visualization based on the collected data, monitor patients at home via audio and video streaming and notifications being sent to the family or physician.

Wearable devices and home health monitoring devices assisting patients are a common thing now. Such healthcare devices as insulin pumps, defibrillators, scales, CPAP machines, cardiac monitoring devices and oxygen tanks are now connected in the IoT to ensure remote monitoring, providing patients and their caregivers with valuable real-time information. These wearable devices, for example, can immediately send out alerts for emergency medical help. Fitness bands, even though marketed as "wellness solutions" rather than medical devices, can take vital data from the body throughout the day and transmit it wirelessly to computers, smartphones or tablets. Moreover, some medical device manufacturers already offer a cloud-based platform that enables wireless transfer, storage and display of clinical data [16, 17]. These platforms also provide interoperability with a variety of medical devices and apps and generate an enormous amount of clinical data which can help the healthcare industry in doing research.

Recent studies suggest that IoT-based medical devices and systems can get patients out of the hospital more quickly, or keep them out altogether, and save organizations money [1, 2]. On the other hand, interconnectivity can provide for easy data collection, asset management, OTA updates and device remote control and monitoring. Doctors and other health monitoring personnel, like nutritionists and dieticians, are also taking advantage of these smart devices to keep an eye on their patients. With tons of new healthcare technology start-ups, IoT is rapidly revolutionizing the healthcare industry.

2.3 Literature Survey

In recent research, various diseases due to the environment, as well as those with hereditary case histories have emerged at a serious rate and need to be taken care of in order to keep mankind safe [18]. To help with this, healthcare management is being introduced as a remote care and monitoring framework through which the distance between the patient (user) and the caregiver can be nullified and precision medication can be provided. Also, in Asian countries, due to the shortage of doctors in government hospitals, they are not available 24/7, and such an IoT-based system is being executed by which a multi-parameter disease-monitoring system is used to measure blood pressure, cardiac problems and different types of fever [18, 19]. Blood glucose sensors, blood pressure sensors, heartbeat sensors and temperature sensors are the parameters used for data acquisition, and then the disease is identified through microprocessors used to provide suggestions. This planned system would be economical for good health management in government hospitals that can be attributed to the utilization of web applications throughout [20]. The studied deficiencies in the system can be identified as there being no medical background or hereditary issues of the patient considered while diagnosing the current disease, or issues like allergies to any medication or food which can be a problem when suggesting a treatment to a patient. Ketone (acetone) analysis can be used for diabetes prediction and cumulative treatment prediction. A FIGARO TGS 822 gas sensor is used to detect the amount of the gas acetone in a person's breath [21]. A microcontroller is used to read data (ketone level) from the breath exhaled from a patient. An associated LCD displays the ketone level to mmol/l and this data is sent to the database. Based on this, three types of prediction can be announced: normal level; insulin required; risk of DKA (urgent medical attention required). [framework1.pdf] Furthermore, the application of the Internet of Things can be used to create a mobile application for a more efficient personal monitoring system. The mobile application can retrieve the data and information from the database and the user can check their health condition in a more interactive display. A continuous glucose monitoring system (CMGS) architecture using IoT has been proposed [21, 22] for a glucose monitoring device. The system proposed includes three main components such as a portable sensor device, a gateway and a back-end system. Human cell study, moisture absorption, chemical detection/reaction and the electromagnetic field study are being strictly monitored here in the case of human body to sensor communication. The power consumption of components and devices is also analyzed to help develop a lower energy consumption system. The implemented IoT-based architecture is a complete system starting from the sensor node to the back-end server. Through the system, doctors and caregivers can easily monitor their patient anytime and anywhere via a browser or a smartphone application. Here the sensors obtain data from body parameters, but they haven't considered any previous case history or the patient's life habits which also can evolve or influence blood glucose level fluctuations for prediction or treatment considerations [22].

Wearable health devices, mobile apps and diagnostic tools transform the medical field by introducing new assistive devices for patients to create communication and amplify intelligence. Secured Mobile Enabled Assisting Device (SMEAD) [23] has been introduced as an end-to-end secure system targeted towards diabetic patients who can't regularly attend health checkups. It consists of three wearable medical devices and a MEDIBOX for reminders and storage of insulin and other essential medications. The wearables are meant to measure parameters like body weight difference, food intake portions, walking pattern and skin moisture that are common symptoms exhibited by a diabetic patient.

Their system also makes predictions using the data obtained from different devices to determine whether there is an increase or decrease in blood sugar levels. These records and medicine intake details are communicated to the doctor regularly using a mobile application, thus enabling doctors to keep track of the patient, leading to shorter clinical visits. Accordingly, the patient can be alerted about the seriousness of the glucose level and thus directed to the proper prescription. In the future, the system can be extended to act as a generalized system, irrespective of the ailment, by adding other wearables in the same platform, or some better version. The blockchain model employed can also be used as an example of storing healthcare data on a larger scale and steadily linking up with various other third parties.

A personalized healthcare monitoring system was proposed by utilizing Bluetooth low energy (BLE)-based sensors and real-time data-processing [24], allowing diabetic patients to manage their chronic conditions. Machine learning-based classification methods were trained on a diabetes data set and showed that a multilayer perceptron can provide an early forecast of diabetes given the user's sensor data as input. Real-time data-processing is associated to the database connecter as MongoDB and the system is connected to the healthcare monitoring system that interacts between the patient and doctor for suggestions and feedback. The data set for the diabetes classification in this study was limited to PIMA Indian women, so it is difficult to modify the vigorous classification model to be applied for different purposes. If a real data set is collected from a real-case execution, it will increase the accuracy of the classification model.

A patient monitoring-based health monitoring system has been proposed [25] for disease prediction, and consists of three stages: the gathering stage, the sending stage and the use stage. A body area network (BAN) has been developed for gathering information like pulse rate, heart rate, body temperature and so on. The specialists are able to see every one of the elements related to their patients. Data like body temperature, blood pressure, heart rate and so forth is refreshed at regular intervals. In the event that the consultant needs to get any information about the patient he can stipulate getting the current health status of the patient by uploading information from IoT gadgets to their cell phones subsequent to refreshing the server. Based on continuous data analysis or input, the prediction can be sent to the patient. From the assessment and the outcome from the inspection, the framework can be enhanced for clients and the specialist to augment their patient's recuperative assessment.

A smart health band has been proposed [26] which is a combination of Arduino Uno, a pulse sensor, a temperature sensor and a Wi-Fi module which are mounted together on a Velcro tape. It has a four-tier architecture having a sensor module, a communication module, a cloud module and an Android application module. The sensed values are displayed on a ThingSpeak channel. The values are shown in graphical format. In case of an emergency, such as a drastic increase/decrease in the pulse rate, a warning message will be sent instantly to the affected person. The project can be further extended to create a whole new system of connected smart health bands so that everyone can be monitored and given the proper treatment at the right time. With more advanced and reliable sensors, the health band can be more efficient.

To expand health monitoring-based research on IoT using Raspberry Pi, a system has been proposed [27] for monitoring pulse rate and body temperature (vital body parameters) of a person with dedicated sensors. Their proposed system provides a precise, low power and low cost system for remote health monitoring of people. Self-monitoring is facilitated by wearables (with display). The system makes use of single board minicomputer Raspberry Pi and IBM Bluemix cloud which further makes use of the Message Queuing

Telemetry Transport (MQTT) protocol for consistent services. Accuracy and cost of the system are equally emphasized by using appropriate sensors. By adding a blood pressure sensor, an ECG sensor, and a respiration sensor, the system can turn into a complete health monitoring system. The network systems have to ensure that the data generated by the IoT devices should be accessed only by the authenticated individuals by involving security controls like authentication by ID and password.

Medical monitoring using different wearables gained a new dimension due to the usage of MIoT (medical Internet of Things) applications used for measuring heart activity, temperature and humidity using cloud computing services. The monitoring and analysis of biomedical parameters (moisture, temperature and pulse) by these wearable devices allow continuous remote monitoring and lead to cost shrinking in healthcare services [28]. The monitoring of the physiological parameters should take into account human body particularities (regions and tissue composition). This is required because the human body's heat and moisture depends on the regions by the tissue's nature (bone, muscles, fat), the degree of vascularization and the tissue depth. In addition, pulse monitoring depends on the tissue's nature, because the light is absorbed or reflected differently on different layers (muscle, fat, blood, bone). The cloud services allow the reading, storage and analysis data from a large number of sensors and patients.

Researchers [29] have done a study to show the pulse oximetry and cardiac monitoring system where the proposed working principle is based on two types of data capture: 1) light is sensed after diffusion through a part of the body – the transmissive pulse oximeter for precise patient-monitoring systems, and 2) light reflected off the tissue is sensed – the more sophisticated wearable fitness devices employ the reflectance-pulse-oximetry approach. The device can measure SpO_2 and heart rate (for a single user). The obtained heart rate values are stable, irrespective of time of the day and other environmental parameters. Also, they match the values obtained from conventional devices, which are accepted by medical gold standards. Here the patient just has to switch on the power button and place a finger on the sensor and the values will be displayed on the LCD. This data transfer is usually done through the help of a Wi-Fi module and this can be extended to any medical system e.g., an ECG.

Next evolved a mobile application-based decision support system [30] using oxygen saturation and pulse rate. In this system, an Android smartphone and a portable and wearable pulse oximeter are used. A web interface created with Microsoft Visual Studio is used in real-time transmission of oxygen saturation and pulse rate values to a central patient control system where instantaneous saving of values to the Microsoft SQL database is performed. The system designed in this work has an important potential for smart healthcare applications that will be used in remote control of chronic illnesses.

An IoT-based secluded HRV monitoring system for hypertensive patients has been proposed [31] where HRV is a quantification of variation in the time interval between consecutive heartbeats. HRV analysis is of utmost importance in recent times, as it is linked with cardiovascular disease, diabetes mellitus and disease states associated with autonomic dysrhythmia, such as hypertension and a large array of chronic degenerative medical conditions. The architecture in brief is scheduled as the wearable sensor will send data to the Arduino module (with Zigbee), that will be sent to database storage or the MQTT server. When comparison and checking has been done, an SMS will be sent to caregivers if an emergency case arises or any urgency is detected. The observation concludes that there is shrinking in HRV time domain parameters beneath the normal range for hypertensive patients compared to normotensive persons, and there is much deviation from normal seen in the rendered graphs of hypertensive patients, indicating increased risk for cardiac mortality and stroke mortality. Thus, the proposed system successfully functions to monitor and provide insights regarding the hypertension condition. As a look into future enhancements of the system, the web application could also be hosted in a cloud environment with storage and the MQTT broker implemented with the same cloud environment.

Research analysis in this domain suggests the use of another portable system [32] designed for heart rate monitoring and warning messages. Sensors are used to detect the heart rate and convert them to beats per minute (BPM) and then save this to the concerned database. If an abnormality is detected i.e., less than 60 BPM or above 100 BPM, then a warning is to be sent to the patient. As a result of the experiment, the BPM average for individuals is based on their average ADC (analog to digital converter) value from sensor to digital device.

As the number of healthcare requests and similar type of disease increase in the population day by day, a system has been introduced [1] that can handle massive amounts of data and support heavy querying. The number of sensors and users keeps increasing, which requires a scalable and flexible system. Hadoop and MongoDB are utilized as the core technologies of the system. There are numerous applications in behavioral analytics of patients. A few recent approaches for cardiovascular disease identification and fall detection will be discussed qualitatively. General challenges or threats to the system like trust issues, security problems, interoperability and privacy issues are discussed. Thus, the roles of government, legislators and research institutions were also discussed with regard to the use of applications for disorder detection and similar advice to the patient. The limitations here are the lack of real-world case studies and limited qualitative analysis on only two patient behavioral monitoring applications, whereas this could be applied to a large sector, like private or government hospital sectors, to run remote monitoring operations smoothly.

A literature survey to analyze the work done by the research fraternity in the proposed field sums up the dimensions of the IoT framework in the healthcare field. Topologies, platforms and structures are reviewed on cloud- and fog-based computing and the security issues to be handled in the computing healthcare systems are discussed and their appropriate solutions are summarized. Hence a system (cloud-based) can be proposed where different dimensions – not only disease, but also life habits and heredity – can be considered to predict their probable abnormality or future disease or symptoms. So if any abnormality or imparity is found in a user or their behavior, then they can be warned, and until they get back to their normal health condition, this warning and medication help manage the cycle. The functional unit of a healthcare management system or monitoring system depends upon the connectivity of the user with their preferred contacts. In most of the cases, the help-seeker goes unattended for a long time, resulting in acute health hazards or dismissal in some of the cases. If a connection could be established with regular monitoring on specific parameters which need attention for the respective user, and suggestions could be provided, the users can be helped with the e-prescriptions provided. In the proposed system, a few parameters are set as they can be considered to be the reason for acute attacks on the user's health if not properly monitored and the suggested actions taken. The users will be monitored if wearable sensors are carried, on the predefined parameters (normal range specified) and as any abnormality detected will be reported via e-prescription generation and circulated to the users, as well as to their emergency contacts (saved during user's profile creation). This monitoring and suggestion circulation will be continued until a normal range of parameters is attained, and hence the process can help the users avoid health hazards or acute attacks.

Here in the proposed monitoring system, some health parameters are considered that are generally considered to be most commonly affected for the patients like blood sugar, blood pressure, body temperature, pulse rate, etc. Nowadays in our stressful daily life and work fields, people suffer from imbalanced diet and unhealthy lifestyles, resulting in abnormalities in these types of health parameter fluctuations or in malfunctioning organs. If proper care or guidance is not given in due time, some irregularity might cause irreparable damage to a person's life, and thus continuous monitoring is essential at regular intervals for users with health hazards or abnormalities. Here our proposed systems give dimensions or guidance on how the system can act as an assistant to users where individual human guidance might not be available everywhere, provided that users carry wearables (sensors) and are logged on to the system for routine or regular checkups. So the problem here is to address the difficulties attained by users who can't avail of visits to health centers for regular fitness checkups, and thus to connect them through IoT-oriented applications and provide the benefits of the e-healthcare system and feedback.

2.4 A Proposed Framework for Emergency Remote Care and Monitoring Using Internet of Things

This section proposes a new dimension towards a remote patient monitoring system under an e-healthcare system. The internet created new opportunities and challenges for the traditional healthcare information technology industry where users and their critical health criticality could be monitored and subsequent actions could be suggested to those concerned. E-healthcare is an emerging field in the intersection of medical informatics, public health and business, referring to providing health services through the internet and related technologies. In a broader sense, the term characterizes a way of thinking, an attitude and a commitment to networked global thinking, to improve healthcare locally, regionally and worldwide by using information and communication technology [33]. Considering these two aspects of e-healthcare management, monitoring and care are assumed to be the services needed by patients or users and that will assist caregivers (doctors or other professionals).

A brief system overview (emergency patient care through remote applications) is depicted in Figure 2.1.

IoT is used here for connecting the hardware interface (mostly sensors for procuring data) to the storage and analytical tools by which prediction can be done and henceforth treatment can be processed. The conclusion can be drawn through disease analysis and proceedings could be carried out either through the patient's past medical history or else by continuous or spontaneous physical abnormalities detected by the sensors placed on their body parts or nearby areas. Using the mobile app, the proposed system creates a notification about any emergency conditions of the patient when they cannot be taken to a help center, and hence a suggestion for emergency services could be provided as a remote service. Also, even if the patient remains far away from the treatment center, through the app the consultant can make the diagnosis and provide services to the patients. Thus, an emergency situation (critical health issues) or predicted problems for a patient can be provided through the system remotely.

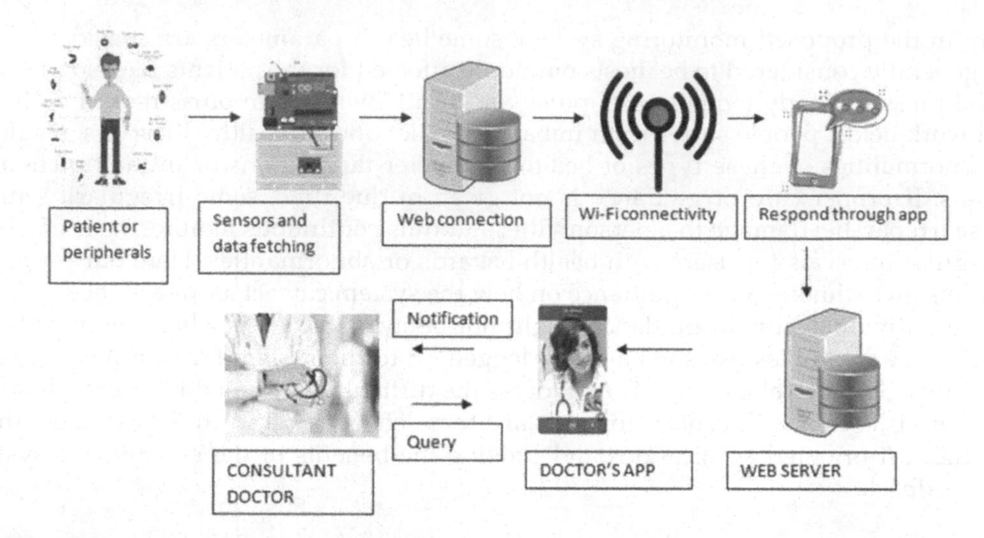

FIGURE 2.1
Block diagram of the proposed system of remote healthcare monitoring using IoT.

Now, for its application, the system may have the following parametric aspects:

2.4.1 Parameters for Prediction

1. **External parameters: (Input from sensors through wearable devices)**
   i. Body temperature (Normal range – 98.4°C to 98.8°C)
   ii. Blood sugar level (Normal range – 80–120 mg/dL)
   iii. Blood pressure level (Normal range – 120/80 mmHg)
   iv. Pulse rate/heartbeat rate (Normal – 60–100 BPM)
2. **Life habits: (Input from user)**
   i. Smoking habit
   ii. Alcohol consumption
3. **Heredity: (Input from the user)**
   i. Genetic diseases
   ii. Family history/cases

Based on these input parameters, the system will decide the current health status of the user logged in and also predict whether monitoring or some guidance is required. The following sections discuss in detail the work assumptions and analysis and sample outputs are also discussed, as given in the form for sample users logged to the system.

2.5 Proposed Work

The following discussion is on the working of the proposed system, with sample data and predictions.

1. For getting input to the system regarding all healthcare parameters, we can use wearable sensors (different types like blood glucose, pressure, pulse rate, body temperature, etc.). Then for connection, onboard Raspberry Pi (or some equivalent) can be used. The last input is to be used as the user's case history. For maintaining or processing these user data, a server support needs to be incorporated into the system. It uses machine learning algorithms for prediction and further analysis to be converted into the user's case history.
2. On the user's end, there is a mobile app installed on their gadget (personal digital assistant or PDA) that would be used for the following:
   a. User's/patient's profile will be created first (like on a social networking site) with all personal information, three emergency contacts (doctor, family members, user himself or herself) and case history of diseases or acute/chronic disease history.
   b. All the normal range data for individual users will be saved against the parameters on the app in their profiles (case history, healthcare parameters like blood glucose, pressure, pulse rate, body temperature, etc.)
   c. At each interval of time (preset intervals), the sensor data from the wearable will go to the app (via the server) from the user's body. When ML logic finds an abnormality (by comparing the input with the standard), it triggers the alarms on the emergency contacts' phones (alarm and text message together)
   d. The alarm label will have the abnormality name e.g., pressure high or sugar level falls or "X" disease
   e. Text message will contain the details of the emergency situation i.e., the normal situation vs the current patient's/user's body's situation
   f. The text message can also suggest some probable contacts saved as the user's emergency help contact on his/her profile e.g., contacting the user's guardian is suggested to the doctor, the user's guardian is recommended to contact some nearby hospital or emergency, the user is advised to contact the doctor immediately or some friend nearby who can help
   g. If immediate action is not taken on the patient, as judged by two parameters e.g., that the patient's abnormality level has been relieved and has gone back to normal parameters or some contacts have been made, then another alarm might be generated to the emergency contacts (not the user again as he/she might not be in a situation to handle more alarms). This can be done three more times at 15-minute intervals until they reach the normal level of their healthcare parameters
   h. Once they return to their normal situation or parameters in which the abnormality was detected, a text message of thanks is sent to all emergency contacts, but not to the user himself or herself
   i. If some sad demise occurs (detected by pulse rate), a text message of condolences can be sent to the emergency contacts.
3. The proposed idea is depicted as the following block diagram of Figure 2.2 showing the activities briefly.

Next, the proposed framework is discussed in sections individually about their implementation and discussion of their effect with respect to the development of the warning system. Firstly, the data input coming from the users is taken as the

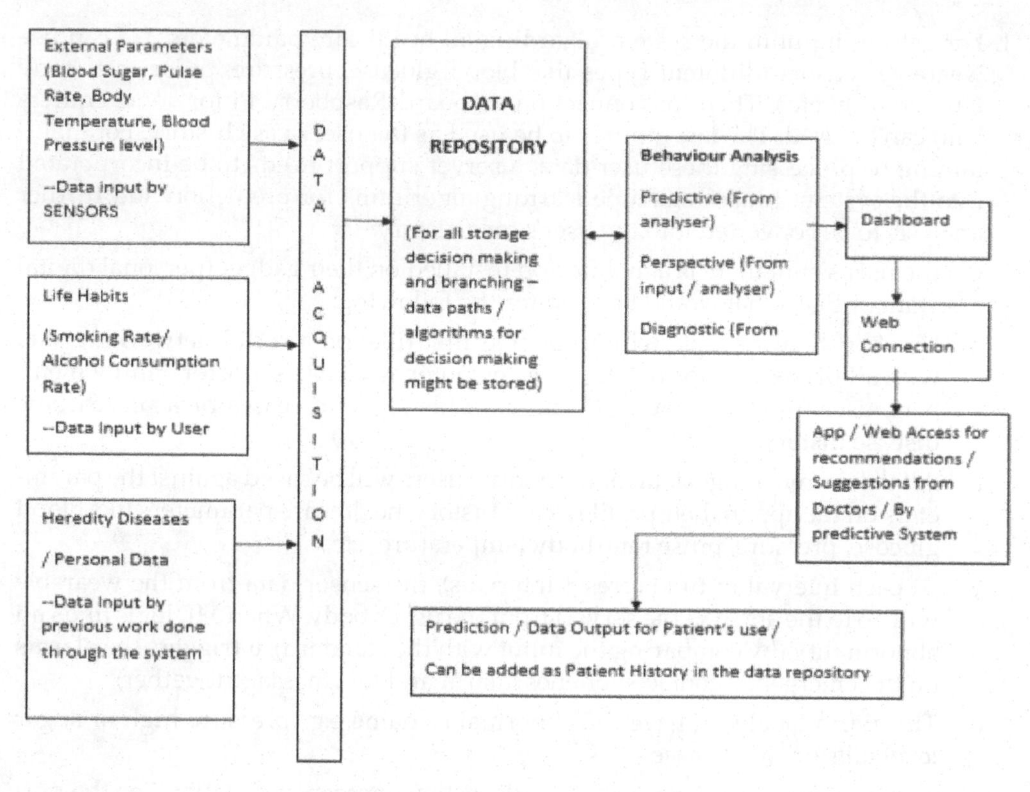

FIGURE 2.2
Proposed system framework for emergency remote care and monitoring using IoT.

data acquisition part of the system which will be stored in the data repository centralized as a cloud storage model.

Data Acquisition: This section describes how the system acquires input, as given in Figure 2.3. It is done generally by the wearable devices, and other than that, the users' case history is also taken as a parameter for analysis or prediction. The data acquisition stage is also all about storage of data in the system for future use. This data might also have the machine learning algorithm applied to the data set so that it can be treated as the case history of a user. The data repository will be allowed to be a cloud-based storage system so that it must be accessible by every aspect of the system.

Data Analytics and Prediction (care): This section demonstrates the data coming through the data repository (kept in the green cloud) that can be used for the users' behavioral analysis through predictive, perspective or diagnostic results. All the probable parameters as well as the prediction have to be displayed on the dashboard (consisting of all connections). From there the data or warning to be sent to the user can be directly connected by the web connection block mentioned. It establishes the client-side connection through gateways and thus sends a message to the user as well as the doctor. The doctor-side (or the app), if required, can take the initiative when there is an abnormality that needs to be sent as a warning to the user. If so, the doctor, rather than the patient, can be contacted with the service and a similar data set will be produced to be used by the doctor, and as long as the patient doesn't exceed normal health parameters, this can run as a cycle of data sensing, acquiring and assistance through the web application. This is detailed in Figure 2.4.

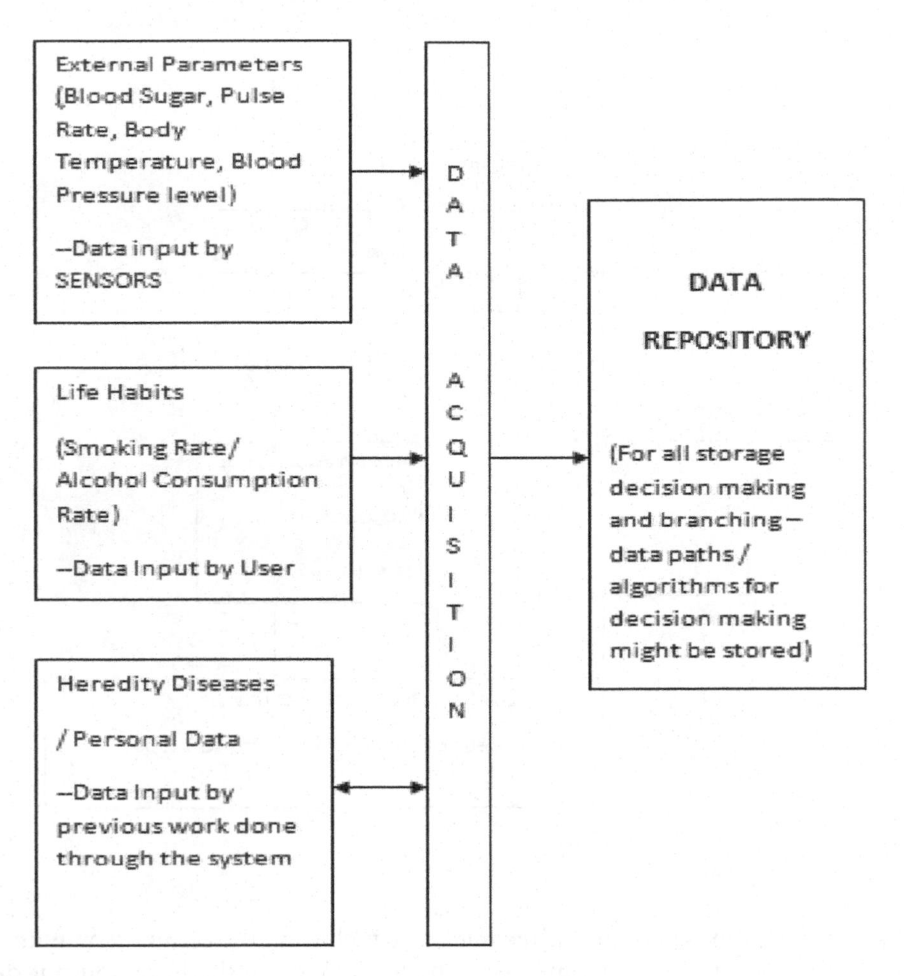

FIGURE 2.3
Data acquisition.

2.6 Results and Discussion

The main aim of this work is to help out users (patients) in emergency or critical situations where they are unable to visit medical care centers often. Here the idea is to consider the users' previous case history and current health conditions to predict whether they belong to the normal data range (regarding health issues). If not, then certain change levels in the parameters need to be percolated to the user as well as the emergency contacts, so that the necessary actions can be taken. The users need to be notified of this according to their health risks at regular interval of time so that proper treatment can be undergone. This needs to be kept up until the user returns to their normal health parameter range.

Section 2.5 depicts the proposed system behavior, including the user point of view, and the current Section 2.6 depicts the input output format proposed by the system by which user data can be sent or analyzed by users' emergency contacts or the system. The data output is not only for sending notifications to the user or to their contacts, but also to be saved for further use as that particular user's case history. As elaborated, the user must get

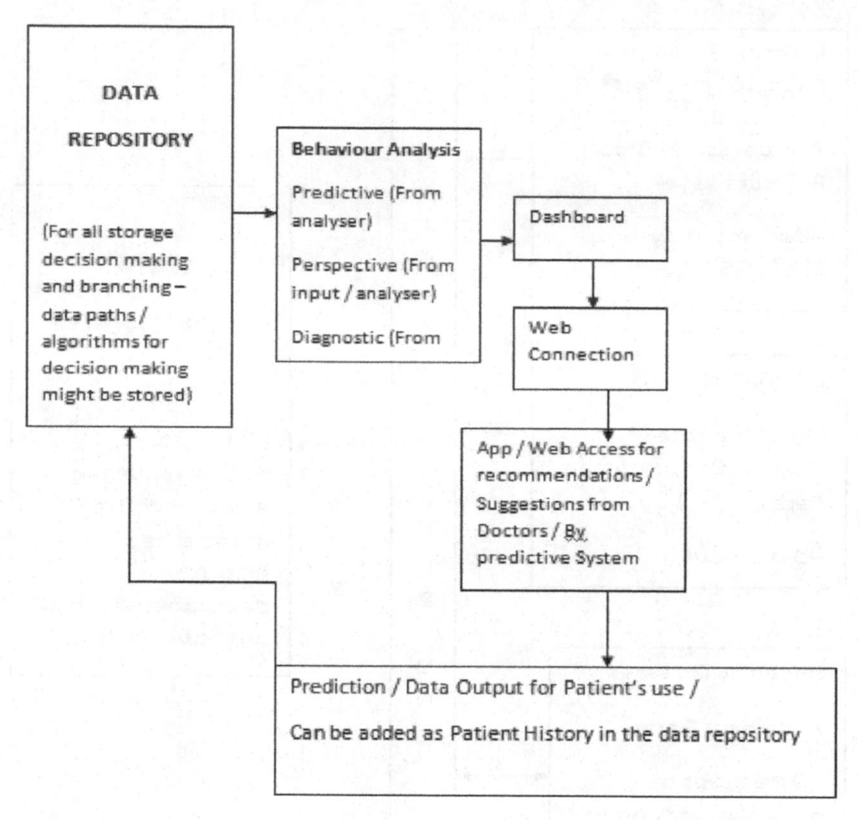

FIGURE 2.4
Data analysis and prediction.

health issue notifications at regular time intervals, including the comparison with normal to indicate deviation from the parameters. The following are the input–output data formats to be used by the system:

Input data format: Input data for the system will be entered from three sources: firstly from the wearable sensors put on by the users, secondly from the input entered by the user on their lifestyle and habits and thirdly, and most importantly, from the user's profile that they fill in as their case history while logging into the system. Based on these inputs, the system has to take a decision about whether the user suffers from any abnormality or not. For this decision or prediction, the system uses a machine learning prediction algorithm for comparing and assimilating the output for a respective user.

1. **External parameters: (Data input from wearable sensors)**
    a. Body temperature: (in Celsius)
    b. Blood sugar level: (in units of mm/100 ml)
    c. Blood pressure level: (in lb)
    d. Pulse rate/heartbeat rate: (in BPM)
2. **Life habits:**
    a. Smoking habit (smoking unit/12 hrs)
    b. Alcohol consumption (average alcohol consumption in ml/12 hrs)

3. **Heredity:**
   a. Genetic diseases (genetic diseases, if any e.g., thalassemia)
   b. Family history/cases (like blood sugar or blood pressure levels maintained by parents or grandparents)

Proposed Output Report format:

User Name: MR. / MS. ....
User DOB: DD/MM/YYYY
User Registration ID: 10 digit alphanumeric data
User Login Date & Time: DD/MM/YYYY & HOUR:MINUTES:SECONDS (in 24 hr format)
Emergency Contact:

1. NAME: CONTACT:
3. NAME: CONTACT:
2. NAME: CONTACT:

Blood Sugar Content	Blood Pressure Level	Pulse Rate	Body Temperature	Any Genetic Disorder/ Symptoms
Normal	Normal (120/80)	Normal (60–100 BPM)	Normal (98.4°C)	Yes: Noted
Insulin Required	High blood pressure (upper limit exceeding)	BPM exceeding 100	Temperature exceeding 99°C	No: Any prediction
Urgent monitoring required	High blood pressure (lower bound exceeding)	BPM exceeding 180	Temperature exceeding 102°C	*
Urgent medication required	Low blood pressure (Care required)	Alarming BPM exceeding 200	Alarming Temperature exceeding 103°C	*
Need to be hospitalized	Need to be hospitalized	BPM below 50	Temperature going below 98.4°C	*
Any others	*	*	*	*

The report tab generated is sent to the user as one health check report sheet, but is stored, and if any abnormality is found, then it is repeated until the user's normal health level is achieved. Along with this report generation, the data for the individual user will be stored in the repository so that the machine learning algorithm can work on it to process future data, and again, the doctor will also get a notification if an abnormality is found in the user. Warning conditions are notified using literal mobile alarms tagged to the system. This cycle of notification must continue by taking sensing data at regular intervals until the user returns to their usual (normal) health condition. If any problem or criticality occurs, then that too needs to be sent to the emergency contacts as an alert message, while the general time interval health report is sent to the user in pdf format as the sample given in the above section. After treatment, the users need to be notified of their normal status and their contacts need to be notified using a specific greeting (e.g., a thank you message), or if some sad demise occurs, a sample text message can be sent to emergency contacts.

Sample output: The following section shows sample outputs to be sent in pdf format to users logged into the system.

CASE 1: ID: User Registration ID: 221NKOL055
Timestamp: 28/12/2019 – 13:11:39
Input data:

1. External parameters:
   a. Body temperature: 102°C
   b. Blood sugar level: 8.5 mm/100 ml
   c. Blood pressure level: 120/90 mmHg
   d. Pulse rate/heartbeat rate: 137 BPM
2. Life habits:
   a. Smoking habit: 2 units/12 hrs
   b. Alcohol consumption: 0.5 ml/12 hrs
3. Heredity:
   a. Genetic diseases: NO
   b. Family history/cases: Maternal parents transmitted blood sugar and high blood pressure case history

Report <221NKOL055-01>:

User Name: Ms. Narayani Maity
User DOB: 21/10/1981
User Registration ID: 221NKOL055
User Login Date & Time: 28/12/2019 – 13:11:39

Emergency Contact:

1. NAME: Dr. Sadhan Kumar Shaw CONTACT: 8958965888
2. NAME: Dr. Drupad Sengupta CONTACT: 7872788922
3. NAME: Mr. Shubhayu Maity CONTACT: 9000529522

Blood Sugar Content	Blood Pressure Level	Pulse Rate	Body Temperature	Any Genetic Disorder/ Symptoms
Urgent monitoring required	High blood pressure (lower bound exceeding)	BPM exceeding 100	Temperature exceeding 102°C	Yes: High blood pressure resulting in cardiac arrest and blood glucose level monitoring required

---

Timestamp: After first doctor's advice: monitoring: 28/12/2019 – 13:30:13
Input data:

1. External parameters:
   a. Body temperature: 99.2°C
   b. Blood sugar level: 8.5 mm/100 ml
   c. Blood pressure level: 110/80 mmHg
   d. Pulse rate/heartbeat rate: 101 BPM
2. Life habits:
   a. Smoking habit: 2 units/12 hrs
   b. Alcohol consumption: 0.5 ml/12 hrs

3. Heredity:
    a. Genetic diseases: NO
    b. Family history/cases: Maternal parents transmitted blood sugar and high blood pressure case history

Report<221NKOL055-02>:

User Name: Ms. Narayani Maity
User DOB: 21/10/1981
User Registration ID: 221NKOL055
User Login Date & Time: 28/12/2019 – 13:30:13
Emergency Contact:

1. NAME: Dr. Sadhan Kumar Shaw — CONTACT: 8958965888
2. NAME: Dr. Drupad Sengupta — CONTACT: 7872788922
3. NAME: Mr. Shubhayu Maity — CONTACT: 9000529522

Blood Sugar Content	Blood Pressure Level	Pulse Rate	Body Temperature	Any Genetic Disorder/ Symptoms
Insulin/Monitoring Required	Normal	BPM exceeding 100	Temperature exceeding 99°C	Yes: Blood glucose level monitoring required

CASE 2: ID: User Registration ID: 222KOL0006

1. External parameters:
    a. Body temperature: 98°C
    b. Blood sugar level: 5.2 mm/100 ml
    c. Blood pressure level: 110/80 mmHg
    d. Pulse rate/heartbeat rate: 95BPM
2. Life habits:
    a. Smoking habit: 2 units/12 hrs
    b. Alcohol consumption: 20 ml/12 hrs
3. Heredity:
    a. Genetic diseases: NO
    b. Family history/cases: Parental blood sugar level abnormality

Report<222KOL0006-01>:

User Name: Mr. Krishnadhan Dutta
User DOB: 10/02/1975
User Registration ID: 222KOL0006
User Login Date & Time: 30/12/2019 – 16:32:11
Emergency Contact:

1. NAME: Mr. Ashim Dutta — CONTACT: 9005236233
2. NAME: Ms. Alakananda Dutta — CONTACT: 8563858383
3. NAME: Dr. Akashdeep Dutta — CONTACT: 7278528578

Blood Sugar Content	Blood Pressure Level	Pulse Rate	Body Temperature	Any Genetic Disorder/ Symptoms
Normal	Normal	Normal	Normal	NO

CASE 3: ID: User Registration ID: 223SKOL010
Timestamp: 31/12/2019 – 18:18:20
Input data:

1. External parameters:
    a. Body temperature: 99.2°C
    b. Blood sugar level: 7.5 mm/100 ml
    c. Blood pressure level: 120/90 mmHg
    d. Pulse rate/heartbeat rate: 110 BPM
2. Life habits:
    a. Smoking habit: 0 units/12 hrs
    b. Alcohol consumption: 0 ml/12 hrs
3. Heredity:
    a. Genetic diseases: NO
    b. Family history/cases: Maternal parents transmitted high blood pressure case history

Report<223SKOL010-01>:

User Name: Ms. Srirupa Saha
User DOB: 26/06/1985
User Registration ID: 223SKOL010
User Login Date & Time: 31/12/2019 – 18:18:20

Emergency Contact:

1. NAME: Dr. Satarupa Roy — CONTACT: 7099253823
2. NAME: Dr. Shanta Das — CONTACT: 7872569855
3. NAME: Mr. Saikat Das — CONTACT: 9005687452

Blood Sugar Content	Blood Pressure Level	Pulse Rate	Body Temperature	Any Genetic Disorder/ Symptoms
Normal	Slightly high blood pressure (lower bound exceeding)	BPM exceeding 100	Temperature exceeding 99°C	Yes: High blood pressure: monitoring required

Here, the system is being tested with respect to sample input data and respective outputs are being recorded. For all cases, generally five parameters are taken as input that includes blood sugar content, blood pressure level, user's pulse rate, body temperature and genetic disorders (if any), and these data are sampled against the normal range of values for human beings regarding the previously stored data set. After analysis, the result is generated in a pdf format having tabular data and suggested contacts. In cases of alarming situations of data deviation, the contacts are sent alerts by the system. In the cases discussed, Case-1 having user registration ID 221NKOL055 is suggested for urgent monitoring in the first report generated, named Report-1, and again after checkup/doctor's suggestions, and the second time, monitoring suggests in Report-2 that things have come under control (partially). In the other two cases discussed, the suggested measures are not really required, as the parameters show a normal range of values (approximately), and hence the problems alone are stated in the respective reports. Likewise, the system will help users who are in remote locations and not directly interacting with caregivers or doctors, but are able to receive suggested measures to take to save these users from severe risks to life or from some critical health hazards.

2.7 Conclusion and Future Work

The work proposed in the chapter consists of a framework for the analysis of e-healthcare data or remote health monitoring and care services being provided to users (patients) who are not able to undergo health checkups at the usual regular intervals. It has been observed in many of the cases in different locations that some of the users may be in an environment where asking for help also is not an option or the caregivers might not be available in their range of help seeking. The system proposed highlights the option of personal assistance as well as remote guidance to the users where they are signed up to the system and carry the required wearables and update their profile with all case histories regularly. A few of the deficiencies have been found by studying previous works. Some extra parameters other than the usual data only received from wearables are also considered to be the root of a disease or symptoms prediction and thus better treatments or medication can be supplied to the users as needed. In this system, the output at each stage is compared to the normal data range, and for abnormalities, the emergency contacts are notified in due time. The advantages of using the system are that it would be continuously monitoring a user when their wearables have data values varying from the normal range, till they return to normal. Thus, users can be assisted via e-health monitoring and reporting through an IoT-based system where the users are not required to be present in any healthcare center to be checked i.e., remote care and personalized advice are the major benefits of this system. At the last stage of treatment i.e., the user recovers or demise occurs, the system sends the appropriate text to the user and its caregivers. The system is still in the testing phase and hence only a sample data set and outputs could be proposed in the chapter.

After testing in the beta stage, the system needs to be implemented through real-time data sets and user benefits are to be plotted against using the system versus not using the system. The literature survey done for the studies included different parameters for health monitoring of any human being, as well as different data set predictions. The study showed different dimensions of security issues and threats for data stored in the system or the cloud storage being used. Not only attacks, but types of data security should also be touched upon while developing the aspects of the system involved. For focusing on the future aspects of the system, development will not only include data storage and propagation for training the system for future prediction, but also ensure security from most types of data and user login threats. The system might be extended such that the user-specific outcomes are recorded for future training and the system performance would be measured with respect to its accuracy of prediction and medication prescribed to the users. If such a remote monitoring and assistance healthcare management system is to be developed and made secure from cyber threats, then it could serve mankind better with each day of its usage via simultaneous artificial intelligence training and management without any further human intervention for disease prediction and further assistance till the patient has been cured.

While a system is being developed for the wellbeing of mankind, there remain some security issues that might disrupt the usual working of the system. Generally, data storage and user security are the two most important parts of the system being proposed here, but after discussion it is evident that there will be security-related problems that need addressing [5]. Unfortunately, the majority of the applications developed through IoT-based healthcare system generally fail to prevent intrusions and other types of security threats. A few such threats are as follows [6]: malicious threat, system or network failure, human error, etc. Other than these, cyber-attacks on the system could be classified as: session medjacking, ransomware, denial of service attack (DoS), which, if not taken care of, can disrupt the service temporarily or permanently. Hence the proposed framework must include the handling of these problems so that the user can freely use, interact with and store their current log as well as their case history for further use and prediction. As future work, we advocate developing a resilient security model to support patient safety, data security and connected medical devices within critical healthcare infrastructure.

References

1. Chui K.T., Liu W., Lytras M., Zhao M., 2019. Big Data and IoT Solution for Patient Behaviour Monitoring, *Behaviour & Information Technology*, 38, 940–949.
2. Dang L.M., Piran J., Han D., Min K., Moon H., 2019. A Survey on Internet of Things and Cloud Computing for Healthcare, *Electronics*, 8, 768. doi:10.3390/electronics8070768
3. Charith P., Chi H.L., Srimal J., Min C., 2014. *A Survey on Internet of Things From Industrial Market Perspective*. IEEE.
4. Pritam G.A., Dinesh V.R., 2017. A Survey: Application of IoT, *International Research Journal of Engineering and Technology (IRJET)*, 4, no. 10, pp. 347–350.
5. Amir D., 2018. Cyber Attacks Classifications in IoT-Based-Healthcare Infrastructure. In *Cyber Security and Networking Conference*.
6. MacDermott A., Kendrick P., Idowu I., Ashall M., Shi Q., 2019. *Securing Things in the Healthcare Internet of Things*. IEEE.
7. Deepti S., Nasib S.G., *"Smart Sensors: Analysis of Different Types of IoT Sensors"*, IEEE Xplore Part Number: CFP19J32-ART.
8. Dan L., Zheng Y., Wenxiu D., Mohammed A., 2019. A Survey on Secure Data Analytics in Edge Computing, *IEEE Internet of Things Journal*. Vol. 6. No. 3, pp. 4946–4967. doi: 10.1109/JIOT.2019.2897619
9. Amit B., Chinmay C., Anand K., Debabrata B., 2019. Emerging Trends in IoT and Big Data Analytics for Biomedical and Health Care Technologies. In *Handbook of Data Science Approaches for Biomedical Engineering*, edited by Valentina E. B. et. al. Elsevier, Ch. 5.
10. Durga S., Rishabh N., Esther D.D., *Survey on Machine Learning and Deep Learning Algorithms Used in Internet of Things (IoT) Healthcare*. IEEE Xplore Part Number: CFP19K25-ART.
11. Damini M., Anurag S., A Review on Approximate Computing and Some of the Associated Techniques for Energy Reduction in IOT. IEEE Xplore Compliant–Part Number: CFP18J06-ART.
12. Tang Y.F., Xu T., Adrian L., Kan S.L., 2016. *Error Minimizing Methodology for Internet of Things*. IEEE.
13. Mathias P., Peter B., Swen L., Horst H., 2018. Minimizing Indoor Localization Errors for Non-Line-of-Sight Propagation. In *8th International Conference on Localization and GNSS (ICL- GNSS)*.
14. Danilo F.S.S., Angelo P., Hyggo O.A., 2014. Standard-Based and Distributed Health Information Sharing for mHealth IoT Systems. In *IEEE HEALTHCOM* 2014–*The 2nd International Workshop on Service Science for e-Health (SSH 2014)*.
15. Albahri A.S., Zaidan A.A., Zaidan B.B., Albahri O.S., Alsalem M.A., Mohsin A.H., Mohammed K.I., Alamoodi A.H. et al., 2019. Fault-Tolerant mHealth Framework in the Context of IoT Based Real-Time Wearable Health Data Sensor, *IEEE Access vol. 7, pp. 50052–50080*. doi 10.1109/ACCESS.2019.2910411
16. Natarajan, K., Prasath, K.B., 2016. Smart Health Care System Using Internet of Things, *Journal of Network Communications and Emerging Technologies (JNCET)*, 6, no.3, pp. 37–42.
17. Sathya M., Madhan S., Jayanthi K., 2018. Internet of Things (IoT) Based Health Monitoring System and Challenges, *International Journal of Engineering & Technology*, 7, no.1. 7, 175–178.
18. Freddy J., Romina T., 2015. *Building an IoT-Aware Healthcare Monitoring System*. IEEE.
19. Rani G.U., Jayant S.U., 2018. *Automated IoT Based Healthcare System for Monitoring of Remotely Located Patients*. IEEE.

20. Sathyasri B., AntoBennet M., Bhuvaneshwari S., Deepika M., 2018. Artificial Intelligence Based e-Health Management System, *International Journal of Pure and Applied Mathematics*, 119, no. 15, 31–44.
21. Ruhani Ab.R., Nur Shima A.A., Murizah K., Mat I.Y., 2017. *IoT-Based Personal Health Care Monitoring Device for Diabetic Patients*. IEEE.
22. Tuan N.G., Mai A., Imed B.D., Amir M.R., Tomi W., Pasi L., Tenhunen H., 2017. IoT-Based Continuous Glucose Monitoring System: A Feasibility Study, In *Elsevier Science Direct, 8th International Conference on Ambient Systems, Networks and Technologies (ANT-2017)*.
23. Saravanan M., Shubha R., Achsah M.M., Vishakh I., 2017. *SMEAD: A Secured Mobile Enabled Assisting Device for Diabetics Monitoring, 2017 IEEE International Conference on Advanced Networks and Telecommunications Systems (ANTS)*, Bhubaneswar, pp. 1–6. doi: 10.1109/ANTS.2017.8384099.
24. Ganjar A., Muhammad S., Muhammad F., Syaekhoni M.A., Norma L.F.J.R., 2018. A Personalized Healthcare Monitoring System for Diabetic Patients by Utilizing BLE-Based Sensors and Real-Time Data Processing, *Sensors*, 18, 2183. doi:10.3390/s18072183.
25. Vijay K.G., Bharadwaja A., Nikhil N., 2017. Temperature and Heart Beat Monitoring System Using IOT. In International Conference on Trends in Electronics and Informatics ICEI 2017. IEEE.
26. Kokalki S.A., Mali A., Mundada P.A., Sontakke R.H., 2017. Mart Health Band using IoT. In *IEEE International Conference on Power, Control, Signals and Instrumentation Engineering (ICPCSI-2017)*.
27. Amandeep K., Ashish J., 2017. Health Monitoring Based on IoT using RASPBERRY PI. In *International Conference on Computing, Communication and Automation (ICCCA2017)*.
28. Aileni R.M., Pasca S., Suciu G., 2018. MIoT Applications for Wearable Technologies Used for Health Monitoring. In *ECAI 2018–International Conference–10th Edition*.
29. Dhanurdhar M., Deepthi R.R., Swathi R.R., Ananda M., 2018. *Pulse Oximetry and IOT based Cardiac Monitoring Integrated Alert System*. IEEE.
30. Ömer Y., Karlik S.E., 2018. *A Mobile Application Based Decision Support System Using Oxygen Saturation and Pulse Rate*. IEEE.
31. Kirtana R.N., Lokeswari Y.V., 2017. An IoT Based Remote HRV Monitoring System for Hypertensive Patients. In *IEEE International Conference on Computer, Communication, and Signal Processing (ICCCSP-2017)*.
32. Muhammad I., Anggara N., Roni P., Era M., 2018. Low Cost Heart Rate Portable Device for Risk Patients with loT and Warning System. In *2018 International Conference on Applied Information Technology and Innovation (ICAITI)*.
33. Avinandan M., John M., 2007, E-healthcare: An Analysis of Key Themes in Research, *IJPHM* 1, no.4, pp. 349–363.

3

Big Data Analytics and K-Means Clustering

R. Sandhiya

CONTENTS

3.1 Introduction

Big data, being an assortment of systems and advances, necessities new types of incorporation to reveal gigantic concealed qualities from datasets that are differing, complex and of a huge scale. Big data begat a tremendous volume of unstructured information, which can't be constrained by conventional information storage devices, like social databases. The collective digitization of medical services data has underlying new potential outcomes for suppliers and users to build excellence of care, improve social insurance results and decrease costs. Inferable from advanced innovations, the report works are changed into computerized groups (computerized wellbeing records or Electronic Health Records (EHR). Since data is in a computerized structure, human services suppliers can utilize some accessible instruments and advancements to examine that data and create important bits of knowledge. Since social insurance information is created in an assortment of gadgets, with high speed and enormous volume, big data arrangements are required to take care of the issues of capacity and preparation. Numerous big data advances are accessible to illuminate such issues. All things considered, human services information should be taken care of in such a way that they can be adjusted for particular reasons. Big data investigations in medical services information can reduce the expenses and extend the nature of human services by giving customized social insurance. Big data in the medical services industry is intended to help with a variety of social insurance information storage, for example, public health, the executives, clinical choice, assistance and infection observation. The healthcare business is still in the early stages of becoming involved with the large-scale combination and examination of big data. With 80% of the human services data being unstructured, it is a test for the medical services industry to comprehend this information and utilize it for clinical tasks, medical research and treatment courses.

3.2 Big Data

Big data is multidimensional and multifaceted and spreads with time. Big data establishes organized, unstructured and semi-organized information that quickly becomes something that conventional database frameworks are ill-prepared to deal with it adequately. Gartner states, "large information suggests a high volume, high speed and high assortment data assets which need financially savvy, propelled strategies for preparing data for better understanding and basic leadership [4]". Governments and open establishments, nonetheless, have fallen behind altogether in receiving big data and using it to adjust the idea of association with the populace. Social insurance, among numerous different areas, is a significant road where the chances to use big data are endless. Expanding take-up of Electronic Health Records (EHR) and Health Management Systems (HMS) has created numerous measures of useful and setting-rich informational collections. While it's tempting to support the expansion of Big Data in the private sector on a large group of refined variables, the way to its development can be refined to an instinctively simple factor – the impact of information. Heretofore the job of information in open establishments has been, in the best-case scenario, remote and optional. Particularly in the wellbeing area, the job of information has been considered to be a result of social insurance delivery rather as an essential advantage for improving productivity and accessing human services administrations. Vital to the progress of information from decline to wealth is the job of data and information – the executive's frameworks. EHR and HMS convey the capability of altogether propelling the crucial quality and effective human services delivery to all. Combined with the utilization of big data's logical strategies, there are numerous ways by which such an objective can be accomplished.

Right off the bat, big data is a tremendous resource in extending the information base and scattering data inside the therapeutic society. Collecting and moving information is basic to information-driven leadership and goes far in decision making. An apparently basic task of staying informed concerning clinical advances at the nexus of medication and innovation can be rendered difficult if problems, for example, absence of digitization, access, multifaceted nature and language interpretation are figured in. Digitization of medical references and writing don't just tackle the issue of access, sharing and language, but with the utilization of computational investigation systems, immense amounts of data can be arranged to prepare sound treatment approaches for serious diseases. Other than cost-reserve funds, institutionalization of care is an enormous positive ramification of such information-driven clinical choice assistance instruments. Big data guarantees large-scale examination of results, designs, universal patterns and relationships at a populace level. This sort of examination helps in recognizing disease outbreaks, foreseeing high-risk patients, counting recurrence of re-confirmations and fixing appointments (treatment requests) to approaching patients. Furthermore, EHRs are immersed with quantitative (lab result and therapeutic test outcomes), subjective (content-based archives, pictures and so on) and value-based (visits record, medicine record) information. Given the abundance of rich datasets that are put away, there is much opportunity for interoperability in wellbeing and social frameworks. The reconciliation of conventional patient-related longitudinal information (drug history, illness list, family wellbeing history) with social determinants of wellbeing (pay, training, standing/religion, residence state) offers a wise and consistent answer for distinguishing and lessening problems with general wellbeing. With such a framework set-up, the patient can approach customized care as well as being a functioning partner in his own wellbeing and prosperity. Besides, later on, reconciliation of frameworks science – the displaying of complex organic frameworks – with EHR information can clear the route for customized medicine, treatment and care that is one of a kind for each patient. Hence, the day isn't too far away when the experts utilizes the characteristic language handling in-order to encourage literary investigation of a person's remedy related to AI expectations; which are produced using that person's visits to the emergency clinic and prescription history to diagnose the nature of the following sickness, alongside with the preventive consideration methodologies. In conclusion, and mostly in a general sense, big data guarantees large-scale investigation of results, designs, universal patterns and connections at a populace level. This sort of investigation helps in recognizing pandemic episodes, anticipating high-risk patients, identifying recurrence of allocating the treatment request to approaching patients. Therefore, the executives of patients, emergency clinic supply chains, therapeutic labor, asset distribution and minimization of superfluous expenses are some significant worth increments that big data brings to the wellbeing area and delivery of care to individuals. Given the scarcity of assets, the absence of talented medical specialists and expanding monetary productivity, the case for the use of big data to search innumerable informational indexes for gathering essential patterns and experiences is more pressing than any other time in recent memory.

The universal trifecta of information, innovation and science lends a demeanor of certainty to the looming big data explosion over all divisions and enterprises. Notwithstanding capital, work and crude materials, information is the very significant missing element for creating yield in the present data age. Be that as it may, there is as yet a gulf between data sorting and utilizing the same for significant results. A change in outlook away from the spellbinding and detailed work of information is essential to surmount this obstruction which are depended on gauging, prescient displaying, and choice streamlining. Any association or organization that is prepared to grasp this move will be ready to receive the rewards that the advancement of science and data offer.

Big data is designated as the utilization of perceptive investigation and client conduct examination, as well as other data-driven investigation systems for extricating an incentive from a dataset. Big data may involve enormous measures of equal programming running on hundreds or thousands of servers. There are various wellsprings of big data. Documentation, business applications, machine log information, media, information stockpiling, internet, sensor data and social information are the most widely recognized springs of big data. The unstructured information is developing quickly when contrasted with that of organized information. Almost 500 terabytes of information are created by Facebook in a single day. Big data can be applied to numerous fields, for example, web-based life, advertising, human services, cell information, web crawlers and space science and so on [1].

Amidst the various wellsprings of big data, medical services associations assume the biggest position in making large measures of patient-connected information which are generally unstructured. The information in human services associations is put away as EHRs which can help in the trading of data among various associations and workplaces. It tends to be useful to make patient information effectively available and usable by an approved client and for additional comprehension of important bits of knowledge by applying measurable apparatuses and sensitive explanatory systems.

Regularly, an organized informational collection X comprises information like X1, X2, …, Xm portrayed by the highlights x1, x2, …, xn, where m is the quantity of things and n is the quantity of highlights. Along these lines, X = {X1, X2, …, Xm} = {xij, i = 1, …, m, j = 1, …, n}, where xij is the jth included estimation of the ith object. Due to big data, m and n are sufficiently large. On the off-chance that the quantity of highlights n is high, the information is known as high-dimensional information. The clustering of high-dimensional information is valuable, tackling dimensionality decrease just as representation issues [1, 2]. Big data carries new difficulties to information mining since huge volumes and various assortments must be considered.

The regular strategies and instruments for information preparation and examination can't oversee such measures of information, regardless of whether amazing PC clusters are utilized. To investigate big data, numerous new information mining and AI calculations as innovations have been created. Along these lines, big data doesn't just yield new information types and capacity instruments, but in addition, new strategies for examination. When managing big data, an information grouping issue is one of the most significant issues. Regular informational collections, particularly large informational indexes, comprise certain groupings and it is important to find the groupings. Clustering strategies have been applied to numerous significant issues [3], for instance, to find social insurance ideas in patient records, to take out copy sections in address records, to distinguish new classes of stars in galactic information, to separate information into bundles that are important or helpful, to group a huge number of archives or site pages. To address these applications, and numerous others, an assortment of grouping calculations has been created. There are a few impediments in the current grouping techniques; most calculations require examining the informational collection a few times, and in this manner they are unacceptable for big data grouping. There are a great many uses wherein extremely large informational indexes should be investigated, but they are too huge to be handled by customary grouping techniques. With the k-implies method and its modifications, one of the most mainstream grouping strategies is k-implies. At first, the number k of wanted clusters is chosen and introductory estimations of group focuses are relegated. At that point, every item of datum is allotted to the group with the nearest focuses and new communities for each group are calculated. The means are rehashed iteratively until the stop or union measure is satisfied. The assembly standard can be founded on the squared error (mean distinction between the cluster focuses and the things doled out to the groups). The stop standard can be a high number of cycle steps. Over the previous years, different augmentations of the old-style k-implies calculation have been created, for instance, portion k-implies [4], circular k-implies [5], Minkowski metric weighted k-implies [6], fluffy c-implies [7] and so forth. Most of them are modified to accelerate counts or for specific assignments. Because of its low computational expense and effectively parallelized procedure, the old-style k-implies calculation is outstanding for its efficiency in grouping enormous informational indexes; however, some modifications of k-implies are presented as very specific apparatuses for huge information examination. In Salai et al. [8], the X-implies technique has been proposed to expand k-implies with efficient estimation of the quantity of groups. Here, the quantity of groups is upgraded, utilizing the Bayesian data measure. The old-style k-implies clustering was intended for taking care of a single-see information grouping issue. In Pearson et al. [9], another strong multi-see k-implies grouping strategy was proposed to coordinate heterogeneous highlights for grouping. Some k-implies modifications for stream information are presented [10]. The gushing k-implies calculation for well-clusterable information is distributed in Banaee et al. [11]. The primary k-implies issue is the situation where the data are too enormous to even think about being put away in the principle memory and must be reached consecutively. In Jaro [12], a few improved calculations of Euclidean k-implies are intended for stream information. Basically, there are a few simplifications of calculation [11] (e.g., an improved new way by which the calculation decides a superior office cost as the stream is prepared, clearing away some pointless checks, etc.). And these simplifications confirm that the new calculation is progressively appropriate for the investigation of big data indexes as the past one.

3.3 Predictive Analytics

Predictive analytics can be characterized as utilizing existing information about past occasions to place the present in a setting and figuring the potential future occasions and how to deal with them. It can foresee what may occur later on and empower associations with noteworthy bits of knowledge dependent on information, which is pictorially introduced in Figure 3.3. Predictive analysis depends on probabilities and gives estimates about the probability of future results. It utilizes different procedures from data-mining, demonstrating, insights, man-made brainpower and AI to examine past and current information, and create expectations about what's to come.

Business associations can adequately decipher big data by applying predictive analytics effectively. As the volume and assortment of information are profoundly detonating, changing this information to data and further noteworthy bits of knowledge is significantly more important than previously. A development in volume and assortment of information expands the weight of associations. Innovation management groups in showcasing, retail, money, the travel industry, protection, pharmaceutical, social insurance and utility undertakings are exceptionally subject to predictive analytics to improve their understanding of their client for their future business methodologies. Predictive analysis assists with making decisions about opportunities or outcomes before they occur and can be utilized in reproducing a specific procedure to decide issues, dangers and the best course of activities in considering the possibilities in those situations.

3.4 Predictive Modeling

Predictive modeling is tied in with utilizing recorded information to create a model for anticipating future results. It is anything but a solitary calculation; rather it is an arrangement of computational assignments (Figure 3.1).

Each progression right now has a wide range of choices. When joined, they give us a wide range of channels to be assessed and thought about. The key advances are characterizing the forecast target, developing the correct patient companion, building the correct highlights (perception window, record date, expectation window and determination date) and afterward making a prediction (with a predictive model). A predictive model maps the information features (diagnosis, drug, lab after-effects) of the patient to the yield target.

$$Y = f(x) + e \tag{3.1}$$

Where, Y = target, $f(x)$ = highlights, e = blunder

The model can be a characterization issue (anticipating if the patient will have a cardiovascular breakdown or not) or a relapse issue (foreseeing costs a patient will create). The last advance of this channel is to assess how great our model is through execution assessment (Leave-one-out cross approval, K-overlay cross approval, randomized cross approval).

3.5 MapReduce Abstraction

Certifiable information is regularly too large to be handled in a solitary machine. A MapReduce framework has two parts – mappers and reducers. Information is divided and handled by different mappers and every mapper manages a parcel. Reducers process the middle of the road, bringing about specific ranges.

Start	Cohort Construction	Feature Construction	Cross Validation	Feature Selection	Classification	Output

FIGURE 3.1
Predictive modeling pipeline.

1. Map Function: Extract a rundown of hazard factors identified with heart infections
2. Reduce Function: Compute the recurrence of each hazard factor

Apache Hadoop is a Java usage of MapReduce, in light of a non-cyclic information stream from stable stockpiling to stable stockpiling. Hadoop ensures adaptation to a non-critical failure by utilizing a plate with the goal of keeping information and a moderate outcome in stable stockpiling, and runtime can choose where to run assignments and naturally recoup from disappointments. Yet, Hadoop is wasteful for applications that reuse a working arrangement of information more than once – iterative and intuitive procedures. Subsequently, the test is planning a conveyed memory reflection that is both issue-tolerant and effective.

3.6 Resilient Distributed Datasets (RDDs)

To resolve this issue, Apache Spark chooses to find a balance between the granularity of the calculation and the proficiency for empowering the adaptation to non-critical failure. RDDs give an interface dependent on coarse-grained changes (map, group by, join) of the whole dataset. On the off-chance that we just need to monitor the coarse-grained changes, all activities can be effectively followed utilizing ancestry. It might begin with some of the root RDD and some changes applied to those RDD, and afterward inferred RDD are created. We can recompute disappointment, since the activity is logged. This is a proficient system to empower adaptation to non-critical failure. This is the key thought behind Spark – it is a major information framework based over RDD. The programming stack for Spark has just become very rich. The Spark center contains the fundamental usefulness of Spark, including segments for booking, executable memory, issue recuperation, connecting with capacity frameworks – and that's just the beginning. Sparkle Core is a home API for RDD. Flash likewise has an AI library called MLib with calculations (like characterization, relapse, clustering) intended to scale to a group of PCs. GraphX is a diagram handling motor for Spark. It can control huge diagrams, for example, an informal organization of companions, reference system of papers, distributions, patients and ailments. Python for Spark is clearly slower than Scala. In any case, numerous engineers love Python since it is adaptable, strong, simple to learn and has profited from every helpful library. Python is the ideal language for prototyping in Big Data/Machine Learning fields and Spark can be imported as a standard library in Jupyter note pad utilizing PySpark.

3.7 Computational Phenotyping

Computational phenotyping is composed of disarrayed Electronic Health Records (EHRs), which are turned into important clinical ideas. The contribution to computational phenotyping is crude patient information from numerous sources, for example, segment data analysis, medicine, technique, lab tests and clinical notes. The phenotyping calculation changes this crude patient information into restorative ideas or phenotypes. The primary use of this information is to help clinical activities, for example, charging, or to help genomic considerations (Figure 3.2).

Patient Data(Input)	EHR	ClinicalOperations

FIGURE 3.2
Phenotyping.

Phenotyping is especially significant for social insurance quality measures across emergency clinics. On the off-chance that all medical clinics send their crude EHR information to the focal side, which can be an insurance agency or a general wellbeing organization, for example, the Centers for Disease Control and Prevention. At that point the focal side needs to total all the crude data to register human services quality measures. This turns out to be troublesome, on the grounds that every one of these medical clinics can have an altogether different configuration to communicate their crude information and the focal side needs to make sense of how to process them in an unexpected way. An increasingly adaptable path for managing this issue is to process all the crude EHR information first, and at that point acquire high caliber phenotypic data, and afterward share it with the focal side.

3.8 Clustering

Phenotyping strategies can utilize Supervised Learning or Unsupervised Learning – information is marked and calculations need to do a "Capacity Approximation", like order – or Unsupervised Learning – information is unlabeled and calculations need to give a "Depiction" or "Short Summarization", like clustering. Phenotyping for the most part use clustering calculations to segment e.g., a patient-by-illness framework into various groupings of patients to help Patient Stratification. We can likewise segment the lattice into various sickness groupings to help Disease Hierarchy Discovery application. K-Means and Hierarchical Clustering are instances of hard clustering calculations, which implies that each datum point only has a place with a solitary group. Gaussian Mixture Model is a delicate clustering calculation in which each datum point can have a place with numerous groups. All these clustering calculations are driven by an improvement calculation (like Expectation Maximization) to accomplish a goal, such as limiting the total of all information guides x toward its comparing focus μ.

3.9 Medicinal Oncology

Something that makes healthcare an exceptional space for big data analytics is the presence of organized restorative information. This is frequently referred to as ontologies or information charts. For authentic reasons, healthcare and medicine have created numerous ontologies for sorting out sicknesses, therapeutic systems, meds, and lab tests, and that's only the tip of the iceberg. These ontologies give us an incredible asset for understanding human services information, such as upgrading/approving all models created utilizing Big Data Analytics apparatuses.

The most well-known therapeutic philosophy is called SNOMED (Systemized Nomenclature of Medicine). It is an enormous diagram of medical ideas and their relations with one another.

1. The patient is going to an emergency clinic to get a lab test. The consequence of this lab test is inputted utilizing a LOINC code.
2. The lab test result goes to the specialist who diagnoses the patient to have diverse ICD codes.
3. Once we have the diagnosis on this patient, we need to treat him with a medical system communicated with by a CPT code.
4. The patient can likewise take some prescription that is communicated by an NDC code.

To use this data, you need great programming frameworks like UMLS (Unified Medical Language System). All these wellbeing information models are imperative to help normal human services activities, for example, proficient protection claims handling. The National Resource Center for EHR Standards (NRCeS) set-up by the Ministry of Health and Family Welfare (MoH&FW), Government of India at the Center for Development of Advanced Computing (C-DAC), which is situated in Pune, communicates to India at SNOMED International. NRCeS aid and support appropriation of EHR Standards, including SNOMED CT, in the nation.

3.10 Dimensionality Reduction

Crude information regularly comprises the request for thousands to even a million measurements. Dimensionality reduction is a lot of techniques used to diminish the dimensionality of the first information, while as yet keeping up the fundamental information qualities. Solitary Value Decomposition (SVD) and Principal Component Analysis (PCA) are two old-style techniques that outline the first arrangement of highlights as direct blends. Be that as it may, in CUR Decomposition, rather than utilizing direct highlights, we test real segments and columns from the first dataset. So it is increasingly instinctive and prompts a small outcome.

A tensor is a speculation of a network, which is a second request tensor. In the extent of ML/DL, a tensor is a speculation of vectors and networks to conceivably higher measurements. A tensor can more readily catch communication among ideas, as a component of a tensor can be very various (parallel, number, numeric). We can have a patient-determination drug tensor which is a third request tensor. A component of this tensor shows for a given patient what diagnosis she has, and what drug has been given. We can separate a cut along the x-pivot (persistent measurement) to get a particular network for this patient. Thus, we can separate patients related with prescriptions for treating a particular ailment like hypertension. We can likewise factorize this tensor as a total of rank-1 tensors, comparing each to a particular phenotype. This is known as Tensor Factorization. It tends to be finished by a calculation known as Canonical Decomposition and Parallel Factorization (CP Decomposition).

3.11 Patient Similarity

In healthcare, the conventional worldview has been proof-based medication, in which choices depend on well-planned and led research and afterward applying those rules, practically speaking, through Randomized Clinical Trials (RCT). The issue with RCT is that it requires a controlled situation just as a populace. What's more, it tests each thing in turn, which is costly and tedious. Persistent similarity calculations use medical services information to recognize gatherings of patients having comparative qualities. Tolerant similarity can conceivably offer an ascent to another worldview called Precision Medicine, where customized basic leadership is suggested subsequent to directing Pragmatic Trials (PT) in light of EHR information and estimating comparability among patients.

Understanding similarity and practice-based medication provides an astute prediction method so as to direct randomized clinical preliminaries and proof-based drugs.

3.12 Distance Metric Learning

Each Patient is labeled as an element vector in X while Y speaks to the Ground Truth Value. On the off-chance that two patients, X1 and X2 are comparative, at that point they have a similar level in X. On the off-chance that they are extraordinary, they will have an alternate mark. This turns into a Supervised Distance Metric Learning Problem. Given Ground Truth Y and Feature Vectors X, we need to gain proficiency with a separation metric d(x1,x2). This capacity will reveal to us the separation between those two patients. On the off-chance that they are comparable, the separation will be small. If not, separation will be enormous (Figure 3.3).

3.13 Graph-Based Similarity Learning

In medicine, we have a great deal of therapeutic information that is frequently referred to as cosmology, or a diagram. Each hub demonstrates a sickness and each edge shows an association between two infections. In the Human Disease Network, we can connect the patients to the diseases. Diagram-based Similarity Learning is an attempt to discover that, given this heterogeneous chart that associates patients to ailments.

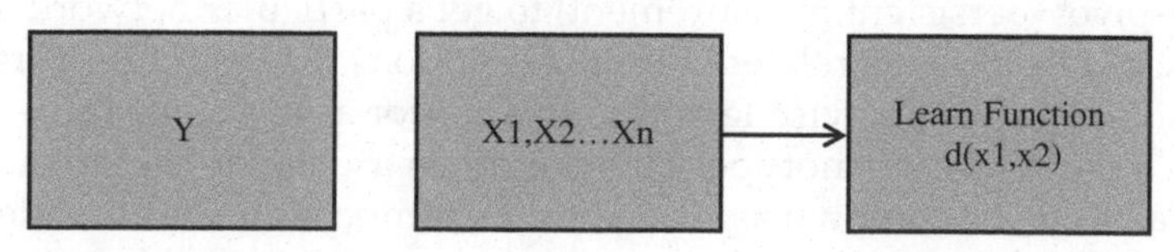

FIGURE 3.3
Distance metric learning.

3.14 Clustering Challenges of Big Data

Clustering in big data is required to recognize the current examples which are not clear at first look. The properties of big data represent some test against embracing customary clustering techniques: Type of dataset: the gathered information in reality contains both numeric and absolute traits. Clustering calculations work adequately either on absolutely numeric information or on pure information; the greater part of them perform inadequately on blended pure and numerical information types. Size of dataset: the size of the dataset has an impact on both the time-proficiency of clustering and the grouping quality (showed by the accuracy). Some clustering strategies are more effective than others when the information size is small, and vice versa. Taking care of anomalies/loud information: data from genuine applications experiences noisy information which relates to shortcomings and distorted readings from sensors. Clamor (exceptionally high or low qualities) makes it hard to group an article in this manner, influencing the after-effects of clustering. An effective calculation must have the option to deal with anomalies/noisy information. Time complexity: most of the clustering strategies must be rehashed a few times to improve the grouping quality. Along these lines, in the event that the procedure takes too long, at that point it can become illogical for applications that handle big data. Steadiness: stability relates to the capacity of a calculation to create a similar parcel of the data independent of the request in which the data are exhibited to the calculation. That is, the after-effects of clustering should not rely on the request for information. High dimensionality: "Censuring of dimensionality", a term instituted by Richard E. Bellman, is important here. As the quantity of measurements increases, the information becomes progressively scarce, so the separation estimation between sets of focuses becomes trivial, and the normal thickness of focuses anywhere in the information is probably going to be low. Consequently, calculations of which segment information is dependent on the idea of closeness may not be productive in such circumstances.

Cluster shape: A great clustering calculation ought to have the option to deal with genuine information and their wide assortment of information types, which will deliver groups of subjective shape. Numerous calculations can recognize just raised molded groups.

3.15 Algorithms for Large Datasets in Clustering

Clustering is a division of information into groupings of comparable items. Each gathering, called a cluster, comprises items that are like each other and not at all like objects of different groupings. How this closeness is estimated represents the distinction between different calculations. The properties of grouping calculations to be considered for their correlation from the perspective of their utility in a big data investigation include:

- Type of qualities calculation can deal with
- Scalability to enormous datasets
- Ability to work with high-dimensional information
- Ability to discover clusters of unpredictable shape
- Handling anomalies

- Time intricacy
- Data request reliance
- Labeling or task (hard or exacting versus delicate or fluffy)
- Reliance on the earlier information and client characterized parameters
- Interpretability of results

Large collections of information containing many articles depicted by several traits of different kinds (e.g., interim scaled, double, ordinal, downright and so forth) necessitate a versatile grouping calculation that can handle various types of characteristics. Be that as it may, most traditional clustering calculations can either deal with different trait types, but are not effective when grouping enormous informational collections (e.g., the PAM calculation), or can deal with huge informational indexes productively, yet are restricted to interim scaled characteristics (e.g., the k-implies calculation). There are a huge number of grouping calculations, and consequently we pick an agent calculation from every class of parceling-based, various leveled, thickness-based, lattice apportioning calculation. CLARA (Clustering LARge Applications) depends on the testing way to handle enormous informational indexes. To ease inspecting predisposition, CLARA rehashes the examining and grouping process a pre-characterized number of times, and accordingly chooses as the last clustering outcome the arrangement of medoids with the insignificant expense. CLARANS (Clustering Large Applications dependent on RANdomized Search) sees the way toward discovering k medoids as looking in a diagram, which is a sequential randomized pursuit. FCM is a delegate calculation of fluffy grouping which depends on K-implies ideas to segment dataset into clusters. The FCM calculation is a "delicate" clustering strategy in which the articles are relegated to the groups with a level of conviction. Subsequently, an article may have a place with more than one group with various degrees of conviction. BIRCH calculation constructs a dendrogram known as a grouping highlight tree (CF tree). The CF tree can be worked by examining the dataset in a gradual and dynamic manner. In this way, it needn't bother with the entire dataset ahead of time. The DENCLUE calculation logically models the cluster conveyance, as indicated by the entirety of impact elements of the entirety of the information focuses. The impact capacity can be viewed as a capacity that portrays the effect of an information point inside its neighborhood. Neighborhood maxima of the general thickness work carry on like thickness attractors framing clusters of self-assertive shapes. OptiGrid calculation is a powerful programming way to deal with acquiring an ideal lattice parceling. This is accomplished by building the best slicing hyperplanes through a lot of chosen projections. These projections are then used to locate the ideal cutting planes; each plane isolating a thick space into two half spaces. It diminishes one measurement at each recursive advance; hence, it is useful for taking care of huge numbers of measurements.

3.16 Privacy and Security

A few creators report that EHRs improve medical services' quality and effectiveness and further the connection between patients and social insurance suppliers. In any case, security concerns must be tended to before utilizing EHR information for clinical research, and other optional usage purposes. A few security insurance components have been proposed to empower information offering to diminish data loss. In some patient information security systems, every patient record is addressed in a table. For every patient, the table has the value that relates to characteristics, for example, name, date of birth, finding and so on. The security systems we examine here depend on this portrayal. The obsolete k-secrecy technique either summed up or stifled credits to ensure each line was indistinguishable from, at any rate, k-different columns. The l-assorted variety calculation was intended to illuminate constraints of k-namelessness. Right now, an obsolete semi-identifier proportionality class, which contained columns of records sharing indistinguishable estimations of non-delicate characteristics, indicated differing values in every delicate quality. A refreshed k-obscurity strategy created for EHR information embraces thoughts from l-decent variety to keep delicate traits varied. Another structure for securing protection has been progressively used recently. Differential protection calculations can give solid security guarantees, yet there are still worries about the subsequent information utility when these calculations add a lot of noise to the information. One case of the use of differential protection is SHARE, a framework intended to total insights on information found in wellbeing data frameworks. An ongoing strategy brings wavelet changes into differential protection to improve information utility by including noise after changes; this can conceivably be valuable for distributing amassed clinical data. Practically speaking, a subject talked about recently in global terms in EHR protection is control. With a conviction that urging patients to visit their own healthcare records will improve medical services quality, a protection system named "Focuses to Consider" (P2C) was intended to direct patients to get to EHR information and helps with creating EHR question apparatuses. To effectively get to control arrangements, techniques dependent on interpersonal organization examinations were utilized to distinguish stable collaboration matches and gatherings from EHR log information and get strategy recommendations. Anyhow job-based access control for EHRs and review frameworks to distinguish unapproved and suspicious acquirements have just been effectively actualized, for example, the AI model to identify suspicious gets to EHR information. Protection is a significant thought in cooperative research. Removal of specific identifiers of EHR information can encourage particular sorts of information sharing for investigation. Ferrández et al. built up a computerized book de-distinguishing proof framework for Veterans Health Administration (VHA) clinical archives, utilizing a mixed approach of rule-based and AI strategies to enhance current systems [19]. Deleger et al.'s work shows that NLP-based de-distinguishing proof instruments perform at levels practically identical to human annotators; however, those levels are lamentably not yet perfect [20]. So as to process the tremendous measure of biomedical information accessible, specialists and organizations need HIPAA-compliant computational situations to have classified EHR information. This is tedious and costly to set up. One arrangement is distributed computing, in which clients can "rent" HIPAA-compliant PC equipment and programming over the internet and adhere to the protection rules. Some open cloud-based EHR frameworks are available on the market. An ongoing access control model intended for cloud-based EHR frameworks awards clients various degrees of authorization utilizing progressive key administration. HIPAA-compliant private clouds have additionally been created to have clinical and translational research information; this sort of cloud likewise has the capability of facilitating EHR frameworks.

3.17 Various Approaches for Predictive Analytics

There are various methodologies and systems of factual examination, AI and data-mining which are most appropriate for predictive analysis of big data in EHRs. These methodologies and procedures can be commonly grouped into relapse systems and AI strategies. One of the key strategies to examine large information in EHRs is AI. Essentially there are two classes of AI approaches to be specific: supervised and unsupervised learning. For the most part, these AI approaches are profoundly useful for big data in EHRs and to make predictions [13]. AI is a significant part of data analysis which is one of the main thrusts of big data revolution. It can gain from information and assist in giving data-driven bits of knowledge, basic leadership and forecasts [4]. With regard to social insurance, AI alludes to predictive analysis models that are refined by the utilization of AI calculations. It is a procedure by which a dataset is investigated to discover patterns and applying the example to another dataset will permit a model to offer a prediction of the probability of a characterized positive/negative clinical result. An assortment of AI called deep learning [5] can help in enhancing the abilities of basic considerations made by clinicians. It can likewise bolster another age of predictive analysis and clinical choice assistive devices that will help patients in the emergency unit improve how EHRs help in basic management.

Banaee et al. [11] proposed an EHR for the management framework utilizing big data analysis apparatuses, for example, Hadoop and Hive. They found that it is conceivable to anticipate patients developing a specific medical condition contingent upon their medical history by breaking down EHR datasets. EHR data analysis mostly falls into categories of AI, associate questioning and patient grouping. From these categories, AI has the most importance regarding secure, helpful and significant data from EHR information. It is difficult and costly for people to investigate this valuable data, and sometimes even impossible. Versatile random forest algorithm: this is a directed grouping calculation wherein the forest is made by various decision trees. It utilizes a mix of order and relapse calculations. It tends to be utilized to predict patients with diabetes and without diabetes by utilizing datasets of EHRs. It is additionally valuable in distinguishing ailments by investigating patients' medical records. Pearson et al. [9] showed the utilization of AI to break down organized information in EHRs for distinguishing unfavorable medication events. Analysts found that Naïve Bayesian Networks are among the most profoundly material strategies for anticipating infections relying upon EHRs datasets. Natural language handling: natural language training is utilized in various associations like human services to tackle big data and to learn from evolving examples in the data contained in the data. It helps to handle critical issues in social insurance utilizing huge amounts of information.

3.18 Why Predictive Analytics and Big Data for Electronic Health Records?

Social insurance information indicates a consistent increment from year to year and the utilization of EHRs has become normalized from 2001 to the present [2]. This increase in social insurance information will highlight the idea of big data. Important analysis and results can be produced from the medical services field with big data. The range of large amounts of clinical and emergency clinic information from open, private and academic medicinal services centers have moved to the big data area. There is an increased reception of Electronic Health Record frameworks everywhere throughout the world that makes large amounts of human services information. More and more articles and analyses address the topic of EHRs and big data. These articles and analyses are considering various ideas which lead to the following stage of changing big data in medical services to accurate information. This will especially depend upon the strength of predictive analysis. Electronic Health Records themselves can be taken as big data and in this way spans the utilization and use of information entered in EHRs. The selection rate of Electronic Health Records worldwide has been expanded by the United States HITECH demonstration of 2009 [2]. Billions of visits by patients have been recorded in an EHR framework for each year in the United States.

Notwithstanding these, there is a high measure of extra information accessible from the EHR about medicine, illnesses and treatment approaches [3]. Be that as it may, people's knowledge helping them to consider, comprehend and process this abundance of information is limited. Consequently, there is a need for PC-based strategies for arranging, deciphering and perceiving patterns from these data. For instance, a patient in a particular grouping of age, race, sex, treatment history, sensitivities and medical history and so on will present to a specific facility with a recently diagnosed condition. Patients in an associated population can be recognized by playing out an inquiry about different patients relying upon their current conditions, for example, individual history and drugs taken. A treatment plan that is given to these patients can be examined by the specialist to choose the best legitimate alternative for a patient dependent on these particular focuses of information. Doctors can have the option to utilize devices for deciding the treatment plans for a patient and making increasingly educated choices about a patient's treatment by relying upon information about a comparable patient population. Doctors can undoubtedly decide fast and accurate treatment plans for a patient through the best possible utilization of predictive analysis by depending on patients' socioeconomic information and medical history. In light of his/her current conditions and observed results of different patients in the cohort, predictive analysis assists with guiding a patient to a superior treatment plan for his/her given conditions. However, doctors can likewise furnish a treatment plan with the most obvious prospects for improving patient outcomes [14]. Along these lines, as the reception of EHR frameworks builds worldwide, there will be a huge increase in the size and assorted variety of information which can be alluded to as big data. To store, process and investigate such big data, social insurance associations ought to pursue additional tools and methods to manage these data. To pick up information and results, predictive analysis is the key strategy for separating important data from the information collected, and numerous associations are using it. The use of big data in conjunction with predictive analysis in the medical services zone is a great force for constructive outcomes in clinical choice help, patient sickness, and emergency clinic tasks such as cost organization frameworks and asset allotment [15].

3.19 K-Means Clustering for Analysis of EHR

The expanding digitization of social insurance data is opening new conceivable opportunities for suppliers and clients to improve the nature of care, human services results. The most recent devices and advances use computerized data from human services associations to produce important information. Associations should likewise examine internal and external patient data to more precisely measure risks and outcomes. Simultaneously, numerous suppliers and payers are attempting to build information facilities to create new patient information. Existing diagnostic procedures can be applied to the huge measure of existing (yet as of now unanalyzed) patient-related health and treatment information to arrive at a more profound understanding of results, which can be applied at the point of care. Preferably, this information would enlighten every doctor and their patients during the basic management procedures and be used to recognize the suitable treatment alternatives for that specific patient.

3.20 K-Means for Very Large-Scale Dataset

For finding the ideal arrangement of a cost capacity with a very large-scale dataset, we typically resort to consecutive strategies. Botton and Bengio proposed an online, stochastic gradient descent (SGD) variation of k-implies [16]. The calculation registers a gradient descent step on each arbitrarily picked data point in turn. Because of stochastic noise, this calculation discovers lower quality arrangements than the standard k-implies, in spite of the fact that it connects considerably more rapidly. Sculley David proposed a smaller than usual cluster k-implies which selects a small group of the information focuses to process the inclination [17]. As indicated by Sculley in his paper, normal cluster k-implies the diminishing calculation costs by requests of size while achieving an identical outcome to standard k-values.

3.20.1 Tools and Applications in the Healthcare System

The human services framework has a huge volume of unstructured data, so it is difficult to do research and make determinations without a suitable tool or procedure. Hadoop is a tool that is intended to process colossal volumes of information, and is coordinated with the MapReduce model. MapReduce can separate the data collection into different sections, each being prepared equally among various hubs. MapReduce can exceed the limitations of Hadoop, as it has dynamic information layer that gives incomparable reliability.

3.20.2 Application of Big Data in Healthcare

1. Customized Treatment Planning: Based on the therapeutic accounts of each individual patient, analyses should be possible, which can be utilized to choose the suitable treatment and medication for that patient. Ongoing examinations will be finished utilizing MapReduce and Hadoop, and following the analysis results, the patient can have customized care designed for them.
2. Assisted Diagnosis: Physicians can disconnect and treat the patient dependent on certain variables like side-effects, therapeutic history and reactions. Utilizing predictive analysis and Hadoop can give data which will be useful to the specialists.

3. Use Review: To help evidence-based treatment, which is viewed as the best type of treatment, a big data investigation of health data is required. The investigation can be additionally improved by getting data from non-customary sources like social and other electronic media for progressively smarter data utilizing big data analysis tools and procedures like Hadoop and MapReduce.

3.20.3 K-Means Clustering

K-implies is one of the least difficult unsupervised learning calculations that takes care of the notable clustering issue. The system uses a straightforward and simple approach to grouping a given informational index through a specific number of clusters (accept k clusters) fixed apriori. The main concept is to characterize k focuses, one for each cluster. In this way, the better decision is to put them however far away from one another as could reasonably be expected. The subsequent stage is to take each guide having a place toward a given data cluster and partner it to the closest focus. At the point when no point is pending, the initial step is finished and an early clustering stage is finished. Now, we have to re-ascertain k new centroids as the barycenter of the groups coming about because of the past advance. After we have these k new centroids, another coupling must be done between similar data cluster centers and the closest new center. A circle has been produced. Because of this circle we may see that the k-centers change their area bit by bit until no more changes are done or finally, the centers no longer move. Finally, this calculation center limiting a target work known as squared error work is given by:

Where, "$||xi - vj||$" is the Euclidean separation among xi and vj. "ci" is the quantity of information focuses in ith cluster.

"c" is the quantity of cluster centers. Algorithmic strides for k-implies clustering.

Let $X = \{x1,x2,x3,\ldots \ldots \ldots,xn\}$ be the arrangement of information focuses and $V = \{v1,v2,\ldots \ldots .,vc\}$ be the arrangement of focuses. 1) Randomly select "c" cluster focuses.

2) Calculate the separation between every data point and cluster center.
3) Assign the data point to the cluster center whose good ways from the group center is the least of all the group centers.
4) Recalculate the new cluster center utilizing:
5) Recalculate the separation between every data point and newly acquired cluster centers.
6) If no data point was reassigned then stop, in any other case, rehash from stage 3).

3.21 Partitioning Around Medoids (PAM)

PAM is identified with the k-implies calculation and the medoid shift calculation. PAM is an acknowledgment of k-medoid clustering. PAM utilizes a greedy pursuit which may not locate the ideal arrangement. K-medoids calculations are distributing (separating the dataset into clusters) and endeavoring to limit the separation between guides marked toward be in a group and a point assigned as the center point of that cluster.

3.22 Hierarchical

In this type of grouping, the data isn't apportioned into a specific cluster in a solitary progression. Rather, a progression of segments happens, which may run from a solitary group containing all articles to n-clusters that each contain a single item. Progressive clustering is subdivided into agglomerative techniques, which continue by a progression of combinations of the n objects into clusters, and disruptive strategies, which separate n-questions progressively into better groupings. Various leveled clusters might be expressed by a two-dimensional outline known as a dendrogram, which delineates the combinations or divisions made at each progressive phase of examination. Issues with progressive clustering computational intricacy in reality: once a choice is made to consolidate two groups, it can't be fixed; no target work is straightforwardly limited; sensitivity to noise and exceptions, difficulty taking care of various measured clusters and arched shapes; breaking enormous groups.

3.23 Density-Based Spatial Bunching of Applications with Noise (DBSCAN)

DBSCAN is a density-based application that utilizes density as the number of centers inside a predefined sweep where the point is a center point. This density-based calculation dispenses with noise points and makes each cluster of associated center points into a different group. DBSCAN is impervious to noise and can deal with clusters of different shapes and sizes. DBSCAN doesn't expect one to indicate the quantity of clusters in the data from the previous application, instead of k-implies. DBSCAN can discover discretionarily molded groups. It can even discover a cluster totally encompassed by (yet not associated with) an alternate cluster. Because of the MinPts parameter, the supposed single-interface impact (various clusters associated with a meager line of centers) is decreased. DBSCAN has a thought of noise. DBSCAN requires only two parameters and is generally inhumane toward the requesting of the centers in the database. (Be that as it may, centers sitting on the edge of two distinct clusters may swap group enrollment if the requesting of the centers is changed, and the cluster task is unique just up to isomorphism.)

3.24 Compatibility Issues

Presenting and examining new healthcare IT arrangements is something essential to consider for the improvement of their capabilities. Nonetheless, this can prompt pivotal interoperability confusions between frameworks. With the significant extension of the executions of new EHR arrangements, we note that the more we create different and heterogeneous frameworks, the more issues of similarity and interoperability we experience. While there are numerous electronic medical records (EMRs), EHRs, virtual products and ventures that are sent to wellbeing bodies, diverse analytical management systems are additionally present in abundance. These last are, by and large, AI models, man-made brainpower calculations, interpreting or predicting analytics [5]. From the available choices, the treatment specialists pick the one most suited to their circumstances. To settle on the correct choice, specialists should precisely interpret the outcomes from tables, charts and dashboards, which are bolstered by the proposed diagnostic arrangements. Figure 3.1 represents the similarity challenges experienced with the coordination of analysis with existing EHRs. The issue brought up in this sense can be communicated by the accompanying inquiries: how would we be able to run investigation over EHR put away information? Free, paid or open source sellers? What exactly surviving would we be able to acknowledge cloud investigation? How can we join Clinical Decision Systems (CDS) to EHRS? The response to these requests requires an evaluation of the essential needs of the healthcare association concerned. Truly, healthcare bodies should move towards the execution of medical work processes, as opposed to the selection of isolated independent arrangements. The coordination of autonomous administrations of predictive, prescriptive, distinct or indicative investigation introduces a poor expense and data management framework, along to a perplexing choice help dependent on numerous yields.

3.25 Different Solutions, Supplementary Tasks?

The computerization of healthcare data frameworks has brought a huge advancement for various partners; from fundamental EMRs and EHRs to analysis of big data, the healthcare sector has developed greatly. However, right now, we note that the presence of a large number of arrangements that react to the needs of big data in the healthcare area has likewise created a significant issue. In other words, the mix of these arrangements in therapeutic bodies pushes doctors to concentrate more on their cooperation with machines than with their patients. Alongside that, having the information and the opportunity to create therapeutic notes, investigate reports of medical histories and include additional actions, can now and again be tedious, particularly if the relevant EHR and its additional items are muddled and not natural. Consequently, this makes it hard to receive new measures by doctors and to connect more activities in each new item.

3.26 Priorities Engagement toward Analytics

The interpretation of medical big data isn't confined to a solitary methodology or model. While interpretive analysis might be helpful in some situations, in others, predictive analysis will be increasingly helpful. For emergency clinics, facilities or other healthcare establishments, the hazard can be available, in the event that they center around independent applications from the earliest starting point, when in truth they have to embrace an earlier vision of what may come straightaway. Various sorts of systematic tools can be utilized Instead of relying use the word depending on the specific situation and the business challenges. Right now, commitment ought to be resolved carefully so as to actualize an interoperable stage, which can gain various arrangements as required. It ought to be noted that medical big data analysis regularly has a predictive aim: as it were, the utilization of applicable predictive analysis tools makes it possible to find a treatment solution before individuals are affected by a particular illness. Right now, analysis greatly affects patients' lives. In this way, starting operational activities by giving top-to-bottom information on the structure and nature of the connections among people and procedures leads to proposing models that create client-focused results.

3.27 Paid, Free or Open Source Vendors?

Executing an EHR or EMR framework can be laborious. Various parameters and particulars ought to be used to create a clinical electronic structure ready to store, process and analyze information in a powerful way. One of the most difficult choices to make is whether the social insurance association is prepared to contribute significant funds for paid EHRs or whether it will just use free and open source arrangements. Right now, studies are run to catalog all current open source EHRs [6]. The point is to give the qualities of every platform and raise the principal issues that cause a problem for their wider use [7]. For the most part, the issues experienced in these frameworks are connected to the regular needs of programming engineers or experts, who will be helping to adjust the EHRs for the relevant healthcare organization. In addition, most of them can't offer interoperability and versatility, because of the overdue combination of big data advancements with their legacy models. With respect to paid platforms, they can be difficult to pick, considering the training size and server executions, and some associations have made a move toward cloud-based frameworks [8]. Free EMRs are likewise considered in certain circumstances for small practices, which scarcely use any smart healthcare modules. As a synopsis, picking between free, open source or paid EHR frameworks majorly affects the advancement procedure of any healthcare association. The era of big data is pushing scientists to think about and choose a broad vision to cover what's to come. Monitoring what these sorts of platforms can give, in a worldwide sense, will assist with having a developing framework that can react to the needs of analysis.

3.28 Data Clustering Strategy

Although the internet is full of information on big data, there is still an absence of systematized data about which strategies and procedures to use for big data analysis. The system of big data clustering is discussed in this subsection. We likewise show in which cases the typical data-mining frameworks are sufficient, and where increasingly refined innovations ought to be utilized. On the off chance that we have an informational index that would be clustered. If the quantity of the data items doesn't exceed m, we can utilize the outstanding data-mining frameworks. Typically, the number m varies from two or three thousand to a few million, relying upon the analytical capacity of a PC. Right now, manage big data. If there is a possibility that the data gathered is greater, frameworks and innovations dependent on equal and disseminated processing ought to be utilized. There are two situations: if the quantity of data doesn't surpass m ($m \approx 100$ million), the information can be grouped utilizing the data-mining frameworks which bolster conceivable outcomes to perform calculations on grids and PC clusters; in the other case (when the big data surpasses a terabyte), we manage big data with Hadoop-based innovations and libraries ought to be utilized for data clustering. It ought to be noted that these techniques can be applied for information grouping, yet also for taking care of other data-mining issues.

WEKA and well-realized data-mining frameworks are utilized so as to show the information of a volume which can be grouped utilizing limited computational assets. A few informational indexes of enormous volumes are created by WEKA. A PC (CPU: Intel Core i7-2600, RAM: 8 GB) is utilized for calculations. The information is grouped by some clustering strategies and the computation time spent for grouping is introduced in Table 3.1.

3.29 The Brilliant Future of Big Data in Healthcare

Similarly, as officials in trade and mechanical areas announce their big data activities have been fruitful and transformational, the position for healthcare is significantly strengthened. The following are a couple of areas where big data is bound to change social insurance. Precision medicine, as anticipated by the National Institutes of Health, has tried to enlist one million individuals to volunteer their healthcare data in the All of Us research program. That program is a part of the NIH Precision Medicine Initiative. As per the NIH, the work expects to

> see how an individual's hereditary qualities, condition, and way of life can help decide the best way to deal with, forestall or treat ailments. The long-haul objectives of the Precision Medicine Initiative spotlight on bringing exactness prescription to all regions of wellbeing and human services on a huge scale.

Wearables and IoT sensors, as effectively noted above, can possibly become involved with healthcare for some patient populaces and assist individuals with staying healthy [18]. A wearable gadget or sensor may one day give an immediate, constant feed to a patient's electronic health records, which enables healthcare staff to screen it and afterward advise the patient, either face-to-face or remotely. AI, a part of man-made intelligence and one that relies upon big data, is as of now helping doctors improve patient assessments. IBM with its Watson Health PC framework, has just joined forces with the Mayo Clinic, CVS Health, Memorial Sloan Kettering Cancer Center and others. AI, together with healthcare big data analysis, increase physicians' capacity to improve patient evaluations.

TABLE 3.1

Computational Time of Clustering (in Sec.) in WEKA Tool

Number of items M	K-means	X-means	EM	DBSCAN	OPTICS
290	538	54	930	5844	N/A
512	80	180	220	2457	N/A
780	620	458	360	4700	N/A

N/A means that computational time exceeds 3 hours or memory problems arise. K-implies, X-implies, EM, DBSCAN and OPTICS are utilized in WEKA. K-implies and fluffy C-implies are utilized in KNIME.

3.30 Fueling the Big Data Healthcare Revolution

Big data is beginning to alter social insurance and push the business ahead on numerous fronts. The adjustments in medication, innovation and financing of big data in social insurance guarantees arrangements that improve patient considerations and drive an incentive for healthcare organizations. Be that as it may, it will require partners – suppliers, clients, pharmaceutical producers, governments and policymakers and the analysis and research networks – to team up and redevelop the structure and execution of their frameworks. They should construct the machine-driven organization to store and connect the huge volume of medical services data, which industry experts gage will develop to an astounding 2,314 exabytes by 2020. In addition, they have to put resources into human capital – IT specialists, data researchers, data designers and big data engineers – to manage this new and exciting field of human wellbeing and prosperity.

3.31 Conclusion

Today human services suppliers, users and doctors create big data which requires analysis to give better social insurance to patients. Patients can have customized social insurance, and to lessen the expense, analysis assumes a significant role. Right now, we have seen the significance of big data analysis in social insurance. The MapReduce model is a proficient programming worldview for preparing such big data. The usefulness of the MapReduce model can be expanded by improving the efficiency of the computation. At present, we propose a calculation where the EHR database can be dealt with effectively with the least amount of time taken for examining the database. The time taken to process the records and arrange the output back to the document is also limited. The MapReduce calculations run on Hadoop groups.

References

1. Han H., Yonggang W., Tat-seng C., et al. 2014. Toward scalable systems for Big Data analytics, IEEE Access, vol. 2, 652–658.
2. Sun N., Morris J., Xu J., Zhu X. and Xie M. 2014. iCARE: A frame-work for big data-based banking customer analytics, *IBM Journal of Research and Development*, vol. 58, no. 56, 4:1–4:9.
3. Wimalasiri J.S., Ray P. and Wilson C.S. 2004. Maintaining security in an ontology driven multiagent system for electronic health records, In *Proceedings of the IEEE Healthcom 2004*, 47–52.
4. Dzung L.P., Chenyang X. and Jerry L.P. 2010. A survey of current methods in medical image segmentation, *Image Processing*.
5. Wu Z., Wu J., Khabsa M., et al. 2014. Towards building a scholarly big data platform: Challenges lessons and opportunities, In *Proceedings IEEE/ACM Joint Conference on Digital Libraries*, 117–126.
6. Wang Y., Chen R., Ghosh J., et al. 2015. Rubik: Knowledge guided tensor factorization and completion for health data analytics. In *Proceedings of the 21st ACM SIGKDD International Conference on Knowledge Discovery and Data Mining*, 1265–1274.

7. Wang F., Lee N., Hu J., et al. 2012. Towards heterogeneous temporal clinical event pattern discovery: A convolutional approach. In *Proceedings of the 18th ACM SIGKDD International Conference on Knowledge Discovery and Data Mining*, 453–461.
8. Salai M., Vassnyi I. and Ksa I. 2016. Stress detection using low cost heart rate sensors. *Journal of Healthcare Engineering*, 2.
9. Pearson R.K., Kingan R.J. and Hochberg A. 2005. Disease progression modeling from historical clinical databases. In 11th *ACM SIGKDD International Conference on Knowledge Discovery in Data Mining*, 788–793. https://doi.org/10.1145/1081870.1081974.
10. Ordoñez F.J. and Roggen D. 2016. Deep convolutional and LSTM recurrent neural networks for multimodal wearable activity recognition. *Sensors* (Basel, Switzerland), vol. 16, no. 1, 115.
11. Banaee H., Ahmed M.U. and Lout A. 2013. Data mining for wearable sensors in health monitoring systems: A review of recent trends and challenges. *Sensors*, vol. 13, no. 12., 17472–17500.
12. Jaro M.A. 1995. Probabilistic linkage of large public health data files. *Statistics in Medicine*, vol.14, 5, 491–498.
13. Burnap P., Rana O., Williams M., Housley W., Edwards A., Morgan J., Sloan L., Conejero J. 2014. COSMOS: Towards an integrated and scalable service for analysing social media on demand, *International Journal of Parallel, Emergent and Distributed Systems*, vol. 30, no. 2, 80–100.
14. Madhulatha T.S. 2012. An overview on clustering methods. *arXiv preprint* arXiv:1205.1117.
15. Weizhong Zhao, Huifang Ma, Qing He. 2009. Parallel k-means clustering based on MapReduce, In *Cloud Computing*, Springer, 674–679.
16. Khan Z., Anjum A. and Kani S. 2013. Cloud based big data analytics for smart future cities, In *IEEE/ACM 6th International Conference on Utility and Cloud Computing*, 381–386.
17. Chandio A., Tziritas N. and Xu C. 2015. Big-data processing techniques and their challenges in transport domain, *ZTE Communications*, 1.
18. Amit B., Chinmay C., Anand K. et al. 2019. Emerging trends in IoT and big data analytics for biomedical and health care technologies. In *Elsevier: Handbook of Data Science Approaches for Biomedical Engineering*, Academic Press, Ch. 5, 121–152.
19. Modrego P.J. and Ferrández J. 2004. Depression in Patients With Mild Cognitive Impairment Increases the Risk of Developing Dementia of Alzheimer Type: A Prospective Cohort Study. *Arch Neurol*, vol. 61, no. 8, 1290–1293. doi:10.1001/archneur.61.8.1290.
20. Deleger L., Li Q. Lingren, T., Kaiser, M., Molnar, K., Stoutenborough, L., Kouril, M., Marsolo, K. and Solti, I. 2012. Building Gold Standard Corpora for Medical Natural Language Processing Tasks.AMIA ... Annual Symposium proceedings/AMIA Symposium. *AMIA Symposium*, 144–153.

4

Machine Learning-Based Rapid Prediction of Sudden Cardiac Death (SCD) Using Precise Statistical Features of Heart Rate Variability for Single Lead ECG Signal

Prakash Banerjee

CONTENTS

4.1 Introduction

Sudden cardiac death is a sudden, unexpected death caused by change in the heart rhythm. Abrupt loss of consciousness within one hour indicates sudden cardiac death (SCD) [1,2]. It occurs when the electrical system of the heart malfunctions and suddenly becomes very irregular. The ventricles may vibrate and blood does not reach the body. Death follows, unless emergency treatment is begun immediately. Sudden cardiac death is the largest cause of natural death in the United States, causing more than 300,000 casualties per year [3]. As per WHO census statistics, approximately 4280 out of every 100,000people die every year from SCD in India alone [3]. Most sudden cardiac deaths are caused by abnormal heart rhythms called arrhythmias. The prime cause of sudden cardiac death is ventricular fibrillation, which creates an abnormal, unstable firing of impulses from the ventricles. As a result, the heart is unable to pump blood, and death will occur within minutes, if it is untreated. There are different types of symptoms of SCD, such as chest pain, heart palpitation, irregular heartbeats and shortness of breath.

The present age is fully dependent on automation systems. Feature extraction and machine learning is the part of automation. Feature extraction mainly helps to reduce the size of the data from a large set of data. Generally, the feature extraction process is informative and also non-redundant. This algorithm helps to reduce dimensionality also. In this proposed work, around 600 statistical features have already been incorporated for obtaining performance parameter. In machine learning and statistics, classification is a supervised learning approach in which the computer program learns from the data input given to it and then uses this to classify new observations [4]. A classification model attempts to discretely classify two sets of data. Classification also predicts categorical class labels or classifies data based on the training set and the values of classifying attributes and uses it in classifying new data. Classification models include logistic regression, decision tree, random forest, gradient-boosted tree, Naive Bayes, artificial neural network (ANN) and support vector machine (SVM). In this proposed method, five normal and five abnormal ECG datasets were selected from the Massachusetts Institute of Technology-Beth Israel hospital (MIT-BIH) sudden cardiac database. The preprocessing of the signals includes a filtration process. Here, the unwanted noise of the ECG signal is suppressed by a band-pass filter. Next, biological and statistical features, such as R-R and the Q-T interval, are calculated. After that, SVM and a logistic regression prediction methodology are both applied for obtaining statistical features for SCD analysis. Generally, logistic regression works when the data are linearly separable. There are a few steps for performing a logistic regression process, such as scatter plotting, which indicates whether it is linear or polynomial. Then model selection is accomplished. After that the model is trained using statistical features. Next, the predicted output is obtained using test statistical features. Finally, the classifier provides a satisfactory performance with respect to performance parameters like accuracy, sensitivity and specificity. SVM is applied for performance of the proposed system where there is no clear linear boundary of the group of data. In the case of SVM, n-number of statistical features are separated by choosing the perfect hyperplane. A maximum margin classifier concept is needed for choosing the perfect hyperplane. A maximum margin classifier helps to provide the optimal solution of a hyperplane from a set of possible solutions. The optimal solution of the hyperplane emphasizes the separation of data as well as the performance of the proposed system. In this proposed system, the satisfactory percentage of error parameter for both cases will indicate the certainty of sudden cardiac death (SCD).

Thus, this chapter proposes a system that shows a minimal percentage of error parameter for both cases indicating the certainty of sudden cardiac death (SCD). Section 4.1 introduces the problem, with a literature survey in Section 4.2. The standard nature of an ECG signal is detailed in Section 4.3, while methodology is proposed and detailed in Section 4.4, and results are represented in Section 4.5. The chapter closes with a conclusion and future scope in Section 4.6.

4.2 Literature Survey

Heart disease has become a major public health issue with increased prevalence in both Asia and Western countries. Research fraternities in both the medical and engineering domains are working on not only giving treatment, but also on measures for early detection. This section puts together a survey of some important works. There are so many prominent works which have already been accomplished regarding this disease. In one work [5], prediction of sudden cardiac death at an early stage is presented, where it is predicted before its occurrence, which may help to save the life of the patient. In another work [6],cardiac disease classification using total variation denoising and Morlet continuous wavelet transformation of the ECG signal was presented, where a cardiac disease diagnosis system built using logistic regression with features extracted from a Morlet continuous wavelet transform for 10 sec and an automated system was found to be successful in detecting the presence of cardiac diseases. Prediction of ventricular tachycardia using morphological features of an ECG signal was established [7] where an algorithm that predicts VT (ventricular tachycardia) using morphological features of electrical activity obtained from an ECG. Here, changes in T wave, ST segment, Q-T interval and number of premature ventricular complexes were considered effective indicators of VT. In one work [8], detection of cardiac arrhythmia was done by using a time domain technique on a heartrate variability signal where supraventricular arrhythmia is detected using statistical features. Cardiac arrhythmia [9] detection was achieved using linear and nonlinear features in the wave let transform domain where extracted features from the HRV signal are used to train and test the support vector machine. In another type of work [10], arrhythmia detection and classification base on single beat ECG analysis is presented. In one work [11], an automated diagnosis of cardiac health from an ECG signal through principal component analysis is presented. Comparison of a real-time classification system [12] for arrhythmia detection on an Android-based mobile device is established where a real-time Android mobile device helps to detect arrhythmia and real-time classification is also accomplished automatically. In another type of work [13], a DWT-based feature extraction from an ECG signal is presented where a neuro-fuzzy network helps to provide heartbeat classification on the basis of the ECG waveform. In another type of work [14], detecting and classifying ECG abnormalities using multi-model methods is established where the abnormal peaks are classified to identify the abnormality of the ECG signal using data acquisition, preprocessing and feature extraction. In one work [15], detecting abnormal ECG signals utilizing wavelet transform and standard deviation is presented where wavelet transform, standard deviation and variable threshold are included for achieving 100% accuracy in identifying ECG signal peaks and heartbeats as well as identifying the standard deviation. In another type work [16], detection of ECG features using wavelets is established where features of small variation in the ECG signal with time-varying morphological characteristics are extracted by signal processing method. Until now there have been quite a few approaches for sudden cardiac death detection using heart rate variability whose biological features were directly incorporated into a machine, but the novelty of this work is the extraction of statistical features which will help to reduce the dimensionality and measure the central tendency, dispersion of the data and provide high-level compressed representation within the internal heartbeat features, especially R-R interval and Q-T interval. This proposed system will be applicable for a single-lead ECG signal which is comfortable, portable, non-invasive and suitable for long-term use.

4.3 Nature of ECG Signal

An ECG is a graphic representation of the electrical activity of the hearts condition system recorded over a period of time. Under normal conditions, ECG tracing has a very predictable direction, duration and amplitude. The ECG is also used to monitor the heart's response to therapeutic intervention [17]. The normal ECG configuration is composed of waves, complexes, segment and intervals which are directly related to different phases of action potential. Each phase is distinguished by an alteration of sodium, potassium and

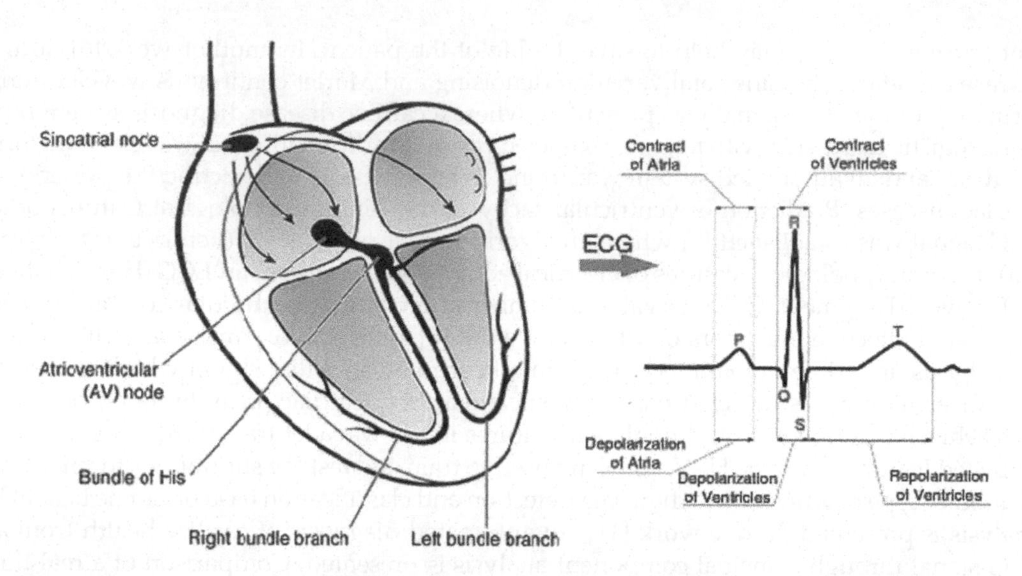

FIGURE 4.1
Propagation of ECG wave.

calcium ions. The quick movement of positive ions of sodium causes depolarization [18]. After moving the depolarization wave, the heart muscle cells return to their rest state to start resting negative potential. Two or more waveforms together are called a complex. A flat, straight or isoelectric line is called a segment. A waveform or complex connected to a segment is called an interval. All ECG tracings above the baseline are described as positive deflections. Waveforms below the baseline are negative deflections [19]. The ECG over a single cardiac cycle has a characteristic morphology comprising a P wave, a QRS complex and a T wave. The P-wave is the first deflection of the ECG. It results from depolarization of the atria. Atrial re-polarization occurs during ventricular depolarization and is obscured, which is shown in Figure 4.1. The QRS complex corresponds to the ventricular depolarization [20]. The T-wave represents ventricular rapid re-polarization. The PR interval represents the time for an impulse to travel from the atria to the ventricles. The Q-T interval represents ventricular depolarization and re-polarization [21]. The PQ interval expresses the time consumed from atrial depolarization to the onset of ventricular depolarization. The ST interval coincides with the slow and rapid re-polarization of ventricular muscle. The Q-T interval corresponds to the duration of the ventricular action potential and re-polarization. The R-R interval represents one cardiac cycle and it is used to calculate the heartrate [21,22]. The typical shape of the ECG signal and its essential waves and characteristic point is represented in Figure 4.2.

4.4 Matters and Methodology

The entire process of the proposed approach is implemented using MATLAB® and Python software and verified with MIT-BIH datasets. A proposed framework for the work is shown in Figure 4.3. This proposed framework contains seven modules: sensory signal

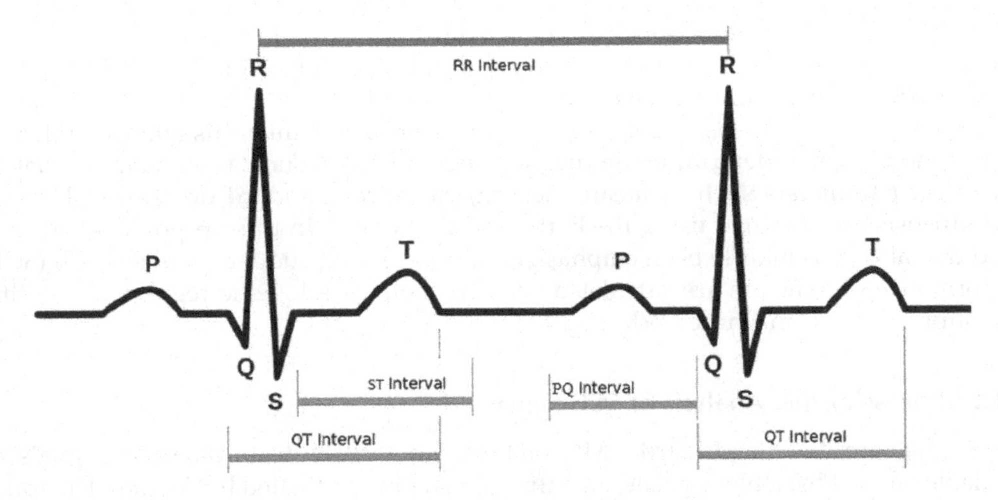

FIGURE 4.2
Typical shape of ECG signal and its essential waves and characteristic point.

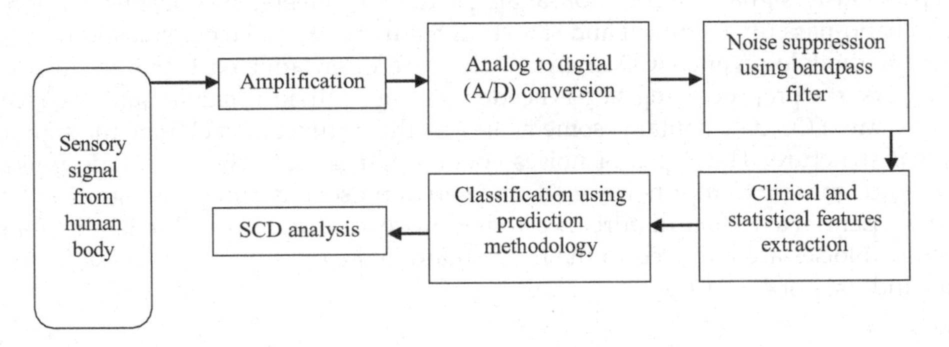

FIGURE 4.3
Proposed framework for processing and analysis of ECG signal.

from the human body; amplification; analog to digital conversion(A/D);noise suppression using a band-pass filter; clinical and statistical feature extraction; classification using prediction methodology; and SCD analysis.

The entire framework is not only applicable to the predefined dataset, but also to real-time data. In this proposed work, the analysis part started from noise suppression using a band-pass filter and the process was completed with the SCD analysis. All the data are preprocessed, feature extracted and classified as normal or abnormal ECG signals which were predefined in the MIT-BIH dataset which is shown in Figure 4.7. Each signal contained around 306,540 samples and the sampling frequency was 1000cycles/sec. The total time duration of each normal and abnormal signal is 300 sec. This 300 sec time duration is divided by10 sec intervals for obtaining the R-R interval and the Q-T interval clinical features. Every 10 sec interval contains 10,000 samples. Next, prime statistical features such as standard deviation are obtained within every 10 sec R-R interval and also every 10 sec Q-T interval. In this way, 30sets of standard deviation are extracted from within an R-R interval and 30 sets of standard deviation are also extracted within a Q-T interval. For finding another set of standard deviation features from five normal patients and from five SCD patients, the earlier process will be followed. In this proposed work, two software tools have already been applied, one is MATLAB and another is Python. MATLAB helps to determine the dataset of R-R intervals and Q-T intervals and Python helps to determine internal statistical features such as standard deviation. Statistical parameters such as mean, median, variance, standard deviation, skewness and kurtosis are obtained using the Python software tool. In this proposed work, standard deviation has mainly been emphasized for predicting sudden cardiac death (SCD). Performance parameters are calculated with the help of a logistic regression classifier and support vector machine (SVM).

4.4.1 Processing and Analysis of ECG Signal

The signals are downloaded from MIT-BIH sudden cardiac death database. Signals are available on the PhysioNet website, an online signal library created by doctors. The source for the important diagnostic information of ECG signal is cardiology. ECG signals are quasi-periodic and of relatively low amplitude and millivolts in nature. The overall process of the ECG signal processing and analysis comprises the following phases, as indicated previously: signal amplification; analog to digital conversion(A/D);noise suppression using a band-pass filter, clinical and statistical feature extraction; classification using prediction methodology; and SCD analysis. They are often affected by noise. In this proposed work, the preprocessing step is needed for improving the signal quality concerned. Basically, raw ECG data contains some noise and this artifact may change the signal from the ideal structure. The types of noises contaminating ECG signal include power-line interference, muscle tremor noise, instrumentation noise and other less significant noises [23]. It is essential to reduce disturbance and improve the accuracy and reliability for better diagnosis. Noises are removed in the linear filtering stage using a band-pass filter which has a band-pass of 4–37 kHz.

4.4.2 Feature Extraction

Wavelet feature extraction is a special form of dimensionality reduction. A feature extraction algorithm is needed to transform data from a large set to a reduced set of data without changing the information. Put another way, when the input data for an algorithm is too large to be processed and it is suspected to be particularly redundant, then the input data will be transformed into a reduced representation set of features [24]. Transforming the input data into this set of features is called feature extraction [25]. A "feature" is synonymous with input variable or attribute. Researchers are often required to convert raw data into a set of useful features. It can also be implemented by automatic feature construction methods. Features can be classified into two categories: local features and global features. Local features are usually geometric or structural, and global features are usually topological or statistical.

Statistical feature: Mean, mode, median and standard deviation are first order statistical features. Variance, kurtosis and skewness are higher order statistical features. Standard deviation gives the measure to quantify the amount of variation or dispersion [26].

- **Mean**: This is the numerical average of the dataset. The mean is found by adding all the values in the set, then dividing the sum by number of values, where n is the sample size and x corresponds to the observed value.

- **Median:** The median is the number that is in the middle of a set of data i.e., first arrange the numbers in the set in order from least to greatest, and after that find the number that is in the middle.
- **Variance**: Variance helps to measure dispersion of the data. It also measures how far a set of numbers is spread out. It is one of several descriptors of a probability distribution, describing how far the numbers lie from the mean or expected value. For example, "zero variance" indicates that every member is the same. "High variance" indicates that the data have some very large dissimilarity.
- **Standard deviation**: Standard deviation shows the variation in data. If the data is close together, the standard deviation will be small. If the data is spread out, the standard deviation will be large. Put another way, If the data allies close to the mean, then the standard deviation will be small, while if the data is spread out over a large range of values will be large.

$$\bar{x} = \frac{1}{n}\sum_{i=1}^{n} x \tag{4.1}$$

This is applicable for obtaining the mean.

$$S = \bar{n}\sum_{i=1}^{n}\left(x - \bar{x}\right) \tag{4.2}$$

This is applicable for obtaining covariance.

$$S^2 = \sqrt{\frac{1}{n-1}\sum_{i=1}^{n}\left(x - \bar{x}\right)^2} \tag{4.3}$$

This is applicable for obtaining standard deviation

- **Skewness:** In statistics, skewness means lack of symmetry. With the help of skewness, one can identify the shape of the distribution of data. It also measures the degree of symmetry.
- **Kurtosis:** This measures degree of peakedness.

4.4.3 Algorithm for Prediction of SCD

Step 1:

Raw ECG signal is extracted from MIT-BIH dataset. The dataset contains five healthy patient datasets and five unhealthy datasets. Each dataset contains 300,650 samples.

Step 2:

Unwanted noise is suppressed by a band-pass filter whose band of frequency is 1–40 kHz.

Step 3:

Time duration calculation of each dataset i.e., 300 sec.

Step 4:

Specified time duration i.e., 300 sec is divided into 10 sec intervals. Every 10 sec time interval contains 1000samples.

Step 5:

Biological features such as R-R and Q-T interval are calculated using MATLAB.

Step 6:

Statistical features such as mean, median, variance and standard deviation are calculated.

Step 7:

Standard deviation is extracted from every 10 sec R-R interval and every 10 sec Q-T interval. Abnormal standard deviation predicts anomalies in the ECG signal.

Step 8:

Standard deviation features are automated using a prediction methodology such as logistic regression and SVM.

4.4.4 Classification

The intention of classification is to accurately calculate the target class for each case in the data. Scientists used to predict the target class using different machine learning algorithms. Basically, the algorithms can be divided into two groups based on predictions: supervised and unsupervised learning. Supervised learning is a process that is based on training done on a data sample in respect of correct classification. Outputs are previously known in supervised learning.

Unsupervised learning is based on the input from unlabeled data [27]. In this proposed work, logistic regression and SVM are applied for differentiating between normal and SCD signals. This technique includes a supervised learning algorithm that estimates a set of functions from labeled training data.

4.4.4.1 Logistic Regression

Logistic regression analysis studies the association between a categorical dependent variable and a set of independent variables. The name logistic regression is used when the dependent variable has only two values, such as 0 and 1 [27]. Logistic regression, sometimes called the logistic model or logit model, analyzes the relationship between multiple independent variables and a categorical dependent variable, and estimates the probability of occurrence of an event by fitting data to a logistic curve [27,28]. Logistic regression is a method for fitting data to a regression curve, $y=f(x)$, when y consists of binary coded data [28]. When the response is a binary variable, and x is numerical, logistic regression fits a logistic curve to the relationship between x and y. A logistic curve is an S-shaped or sigmoid curve, often used to model population growth, and is represented in Figure 4.6. A logistic curve starts with slow, linear growth, followed by exponential growth, which then slows again to a stable rate. A simple logistic function is defined by the formula. A decision boundary is a pretty simple concept. Logistic regression is a classification algorithm which has some decision such as Yes/No, True/False, Red/Yellow/Orange [28]. Our prediction function, however, returns a probability score between 0 and 1. A decision boundary is a threshold or tipping point that helps to determine which category to choose based on probability [28]. For example, if the threshold is .5 and prediction function is .7, then observation is positive. If the prediction was .2, then it is classified as negative. For logistic regression with multiple classes, it could be to select the class with the highest predicted probability. If $p \geq 0.5$, then it is treated class=1(probability is denoted p)

$$p < 0.5, \text{ then it is treated class=0}$$

Mathematically, a logistic regression curve is represented in this way

$$y = \frac{1}{1+e^{x}} \tag{4.4}$$

Sigmoid function: In order to map predicted values to probabilities, we use the Sigmoid function. The function helps to map any real value into another value between 0 and 1. In machine learning, the Sigmoid function is used to map predictions to probabilities [28].

4.4.4.2 Support Vector Machine

A Support Vector Machine (SVM) is a supervised machine learning algorithm which can be used for both classification or regression challenges. However, it is mostly used in classification problems. In this algorithm, each data item is plotted as a point in n-dimensional space (where n indicates the number of features), with the value of each feature being the value of a particular coordinate [28]. Then, classification is performed by finding the hyperplane that differentiates the two classes very well [28]. The smallest perpendicular distance to a training observation from the hyperplane is known as the margin, and the largest separated margin is called the maximum margin hyperplane. In other words, maximizing the distances between the nearest data point and the hyper-plane will help us to determine the right hyperplane [28] (Figure 4.4).

4.4.4.2.1 The Case When the Data Are Linearly Separable

To explain the mystery of SVMs, let us consider a simple problem, where classes are linearly separable. Let the dataset D be given as (X_1, y_1), (X_2, y_2)...(X_D, y_D) where X_iis the set of training tuples with associated class labels, y_i [28]. Each y_i can take one of two values either +1 or −1, corresponding to the classes I and classes II, respectively. From the graph it can be seen that the 2-D data are linearly separable. Here, a straight line indicates that tuples are separated by class +1 from all the tuples from −1 [28]. A linearly separable line is represented in Figure 4.5.

4.4.4.2.2 Optimal Solution of SVM Classifier

There are infinite numbers of separating lines among the data which are linearly separable. It is a challenge for researchers to find the "perfect" one which will have minimum classification errors. SVM approaches this problem by searching for the maximum marginal by hyperplane and their associated margins [28]. It is expected that the hyperplane with the larger margin will be more accurate than the hyperplane with the smaller margin. This is why the SVM searches to find the perfect hyperplane with the largest margin [28]. The largest margin with the hyperplane is called the maximum marginal hyperplane (MMH) [28]. The associated margin gives the largest separation between classes [28] (Figure 4.6).

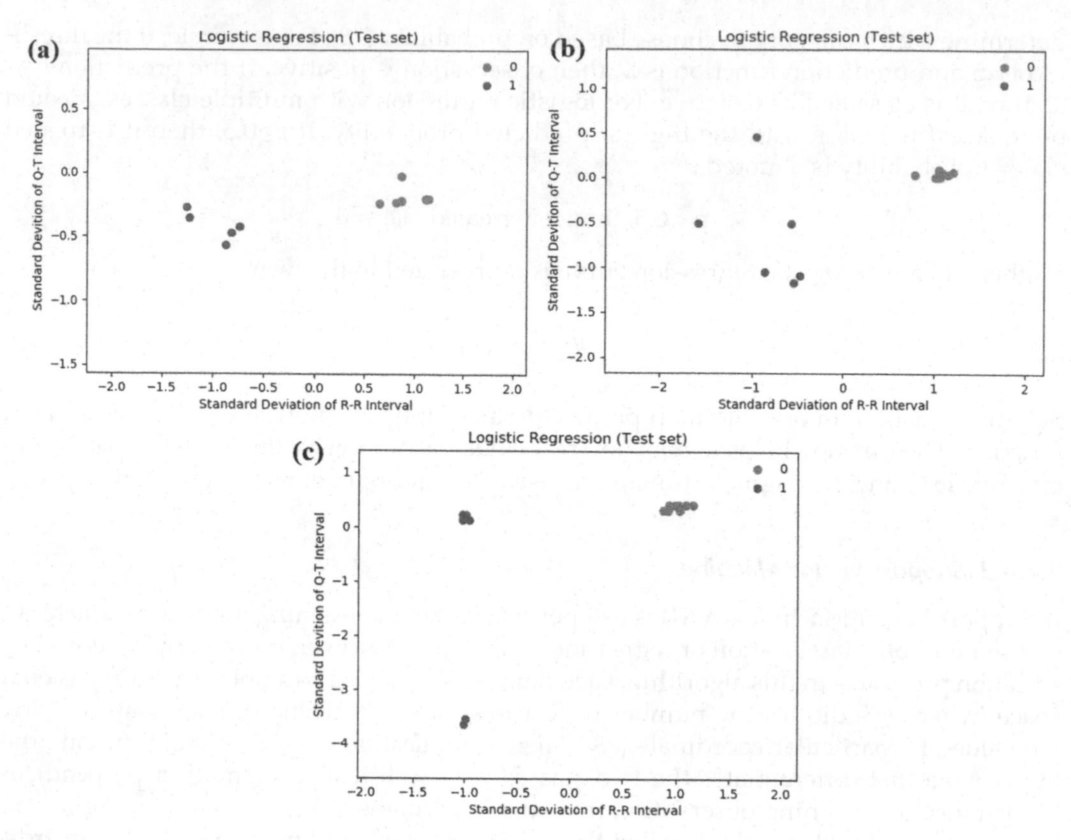

FIGURE 4.4
(a),(b),(c) Test output of logistic regression.

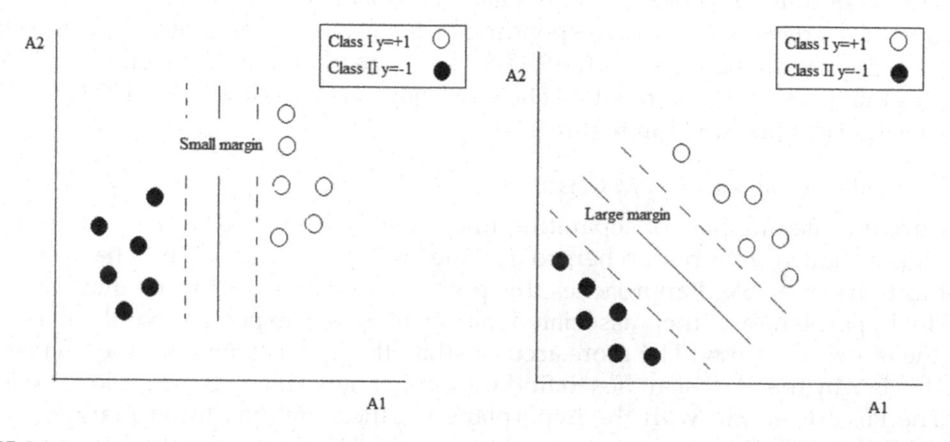

FIGURE 4.5
Two possible separating hyperplanes and their associated margins.

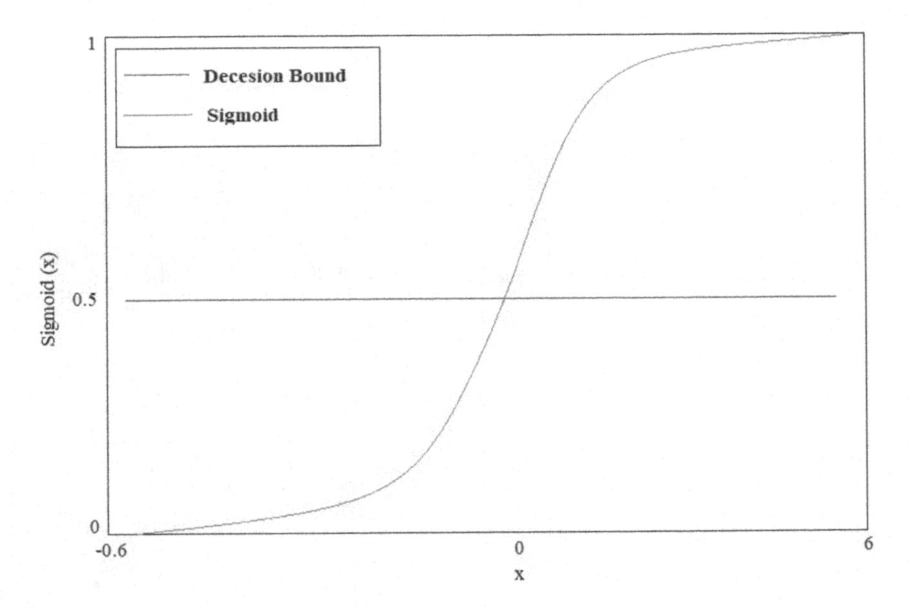

FIGURE 4.6
Sigmoid function curve.

4.5 Results and Discussion

The ECG signal which contains five normal patients' datasets and another five SCD patients' datasets were extracted from the MIT-BIH source. After extracting the dataset, they were denoised using the band-pass filter which has the frequency range 1–40 KHz and a sampling frequency of 1000 Hz. The raw and filtered ECG signals of normal and SCD patients are represented in Figure 4.7(a), (b), (c), (d). Next, it was subjected to the calculation of the total time duration of entire signal i.e., 300 sec. Then a 300 sec time interval was segmented to obtain a 30 sec sample within a 10 sec time interval. The proposed algorithm of sudden cardiac death prediction is tested rigorously in MATLAB 2018 and Python. Biological features such as the R-R and Q-T intervals are obtained using MATLAB2018 from the segmented signal. Next, precise statistical features like mean, median, variance and standard deviation are calculated using the Python software tool. In this proposed work, abnormal standard deviation has been emphasized to predict sudden cardiac death (SCD). A standard deviation of every 10 sec interval split signal is represented in Table 4.1. After extraction of the standard deviation of every 10 sec interval for both R-R and Q-T intervals, values are applied in different prediction methodology such as a logistic regression classifier and SVM. In other words, it may be discussed that statistical feature of around 600 standard deviation values are automated using a logistic regression classifier. The classifier performance is based on a confusion matrix which is shown in Table 4.2. Performance parameters like sensitivity, specificity and accuracy are obtained through a confusion matrix coefficient such as TP (true positive), TN (true negative), FN (false negative) and FP (false positive) from set of classification output [25].Performancematrix coefficient test outputs are represented in Table 4.3. The value of a performance parameter for

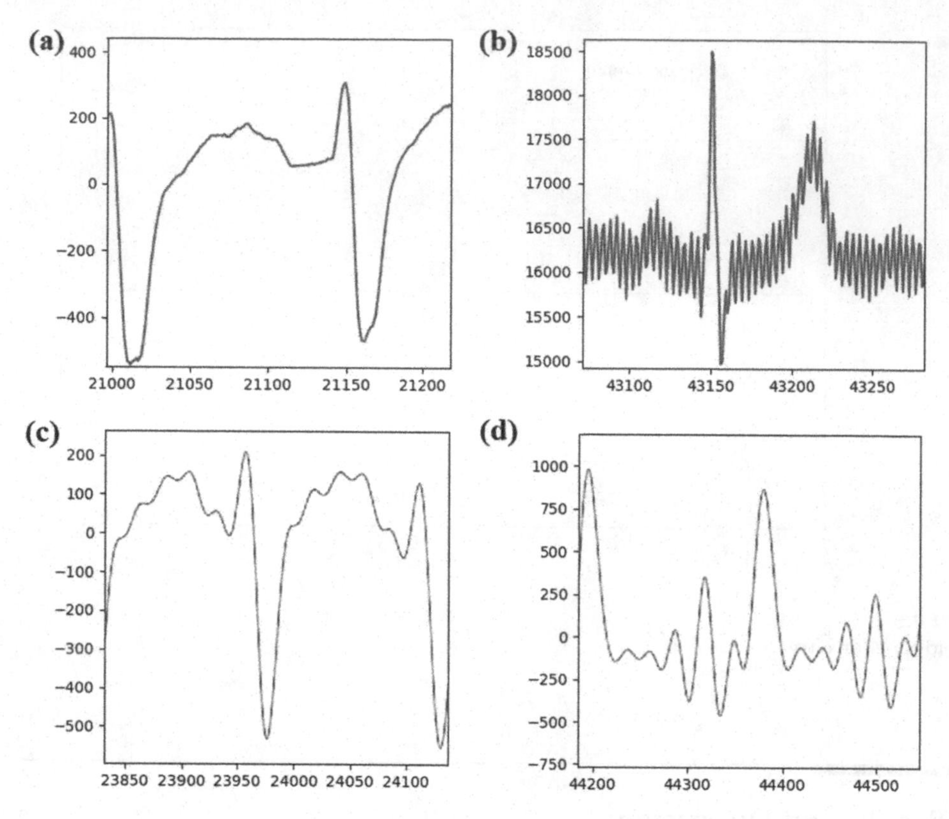

FIGURE 4.7
(a),(b) denote raw ECG signal of normal and SCD patient; (c),(d) denote filtered ECG signal of normal and SCD patient.

both SVM and logistic regression in the cases is100%, which is endorsed in Table 4.4. The logistic regression test output and scattered plot are visualized in Figure 4.4(a), (b), (c). This satisfactory percentage concluded that data are highly separable (Figure 4.8).

4.6 Conclusion

Predicting SCD (sudden cardiac death) is a challenging task without additional biological information. In this paper, prediction of sudden cardiac death is proposed using a precise statistical feature which will be applicable for a single lead ECG signal. This study includes the development of feature classification using logistic regression. This result shows that statistical features like standard deviation are a much better predictor than other common. ECG features. The experimental set of results of the proposed system is able to achieve outstanding prediction analysis. The result shave shown that the logistic regression and SVM classifier both have achieved outstanding performance with 100% sensitivity, accuracy and specificity. A future extension of this work is the challenge to make a portable single-lead ECG device with the respective data and information of this proposed work for real-life applications in the medical field.

TABLE 4.1

Standard Deviation Calculation within R-R and Q-T Interval

Standard Deviation			
SCD Patient		Normal Patient	
(R-R)interval	**Q-T(interval)**	**R-R(interval)**	**Q-T(interval)**
198(R-R1)	38.5(Q-T1)	245.5(R-R1)	60(Q-T1)
192(R-R3)	33(Q-T3)	245(R-R2)	60(Q-T2)
189(R-R4)	33(Q-T4)	243(R-R3)	60(Q-T3)
195(R-R5)	31.5(Q-T5)	253(R-R4)	78(Q-T4)
191(R-R6)	41(Q-T6)	248(R-R5)	61(Q-T5)
185(R-R7)	33(Q-T7)	251(R-R6)	61(Q-T6)
188(R-R8)	145(Q-T8)	253(R-R7)	61(Q-T7)
176(R-R10)	33.0(Q-T10)	253(R-R8)	62(Q-T8)
186(R-R11)	39(Q-T11)	253(R-R9)	62(Q-T9)
186(R-R12)	33(Q-T12)	255(R-R10)	62(Q-T10)
176(R-R14)	50.5(Q-T14)	255(R-R11)	62(Q-T11)
175(R-R15)	57.5(Q-T15)	256(R-R12)	62(Q-T12)
163(R-R16)	82.0(Q-T16)	255(R-R13)	62(Q-T13)
168(R-R17)	188.0(Q-T17)	262.5(R-R14)	62(Q-T14)
167(R-R18)	225.5(Q-T18)	261(R-R15)	62(Q-T15)
180(R-R19)	348(Q-T19)	262(R-R16)	63(Q-T16)
176(R-R20)	444.5(Q-T20)	261(R-R17)	63(Q-T17)
192(R-R21)	31(Q-T21)	263(R-R18)	63(Q-T18)
205(R-R22)	33(Q-T22)	254(R-R19)	62(Q-T19)
195(R-R23)	37(Q-T23)	262(R-R20)	63(Q-T20)
193(R-R24)	45(Q-T24)	262(R-R21)	63(Q-T21)
197(R-R25)	44.5(Q-T25)	261(R-R23)	63(Q-T23)
194(R-R26)	44.5(Q-T26)	263(R-R24)	63(Q-T24)
187(R-R28)	43(Q-T28)	262(R-R25)	63(Q-T25)
181(R-R30)	41(Q-T30)	262(R-R26)	63(Q-T26)

TABLE 4.2

Performance Parameter of Classifier

		Target			
Confusion Matrix		**Positive**	**Negative**		
Model	Positive	a	B	Positive predictive value	a/(a+b)
	Negative	c	D	Negative predictive value	d/(c+d)
		Sensitivity a/(a+c)	Specificity b/(b+d)	Accuracy (a+d)/(a+b+c+d)	

TABLE 4.3
Performance Matrix Coefficient

Classifier's Name	TP	FP	TN	FN
Logistic RegressionTest1	9	0	5	0
Logistic RegressionTest2	8	0	6	0
Logistic RegressionTest3	8	0	6	0
Logistic RegressionTest4	8	0	7	0
Logistic RegressionTest5	9	0	6	0
SVM Test1	6	0	6	0
SVM Test2	6	0	7	0
SVM Test3	6	0	8	0
SVM Test4	7	0	5	0
SVM Test5	6	0	8	0

TABLE 4.4
Performance Parameter of Logistic Regression Classifier

Performance Parameter	Logistic Regression	SVM
Sensitivity(ST)	100%	100%
Specificity(SF)	100%	100%
Accuracy(AC)	100%	100%

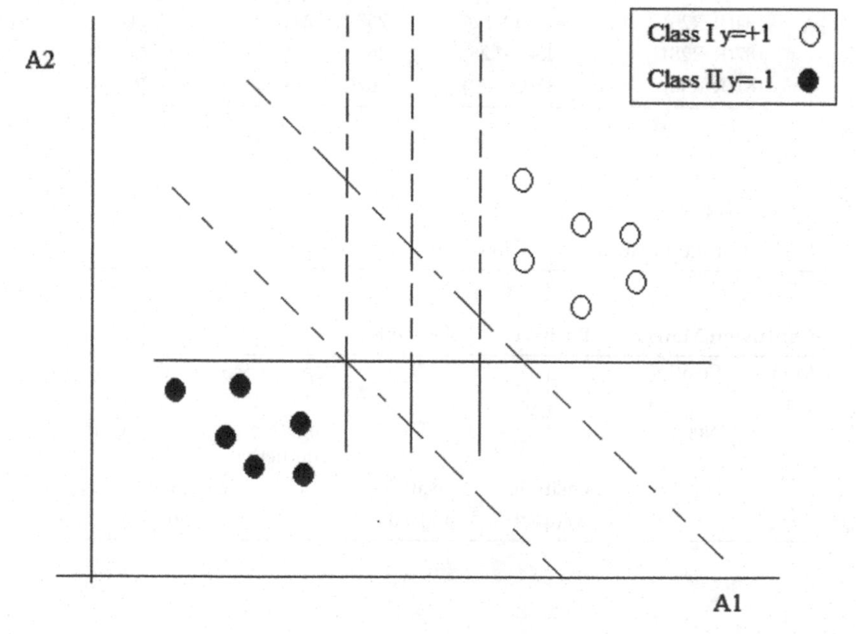

FIGURE 4.8
Linearly separable training data.

References

1. Caesarendra W., Ismail R., Kurniawan D., Karwiky G., Ahmad C. 2016. Sudden cardiac death predictor based on spatial QRS-T angle feature and support vector machine case study for cardiac disease detection in Indonesia. In 2016 IEEE EMBS Conference on Biomedical Engineering and Sciences (IECBES). IEEE, doi: 10.1109/IECBES.2016.784344, pp. 186–192.
2. Vanitha L., Suresh G., Jenefar Sheela C. 2014. Sudden cardiac death prediction system using Hybrid classifier In International Conference on Electronics and Communication Systems (ICECS). IEEE, pp. 1–5.
3. Priya N.S., Balakrishnan R. 2011. A novel algorithm for sudden cardiac death risk estimation using Lab VIEW. In International Conference on Recent Trends in Information Technology (ICRTIT). IEEE, doi: 10.1109/ICRTIT.2011.5972390, pp. 906–909.
4. Khalid S., Khalil T., Nasreen S. 2014. A survey of feature selection and feature extraction techniques in machine learning. In *Science and Information Conference*, pp. 372–378.
5. Devi R., Tyagi H.K., Kumar D. Early stage prediction of sudden cardiac death. In International Conference on Wireless Communications, Signal Processing and Networking (WiSPNET). IEEE, pp. 2005–2008.
6. Al Abdi, R. M., Jarrah M. 2018. Cardiac disease classification using total variation denoising and morlet continuous wavelet transformation of ECG signals. In *14th International Colloquium on Signal Processing and Its Applications (CSPA)*. IEEE, pp. 57–60.
7. Riasi A., Mohebbi M. 2015. Prediction of ventricular tachycardia using morphological features of ECG signal. *The International Symposium on Artificial Intelligence and Signal Processing (AISP)*, pp. 170–175.
8. Bendani D., Berrached N.E. 2017. Detection of cardiac arrhythmia by using time domain technique on heart rate variability signals. In 2nd International Conference on Bio-Engineering for Smart Technologies (BioSMART). IEEE, pp. 1–4.
9. Sivanantham A., Devi S.S. 2014. Cardiac arrhythmia detection using linear and non-linear features of HRV signal. In 2014 International Conference on Advanced Communications, Control and Computing Technologies. IEEE, pp. 795–799.
10. Pathoumvanh S., Hamamoto K., Indahak P. 2014. Arrhythmias detection and classification base on single beat ECG analysis. In 4th Joint International Conference on Information and Communication Technology, Electronic and Electrical Engineering (JICTEE). IEEE, pp. 1–4.
11. Martis R.J., Acharya U.R., Mand K.M., Ray A.K., Chakraborty C. 2012. Application of principal component analysis to ECG signals for automated diagnosis of cardiac health. *Expert Systems with Applications*, pp. 11792–11800.
12. Leutheuser H., Gradl S., Kugler P., Anneken L, Arnold M., Achenbach S., Eskofier B.M. 2014. Comparison of real-time classification systems for arrhythmia detection on Android-based mobile devices. In 36th Annual International Conference of the IEEE Engineering in Medicine and Biology Society, pp. 2690–2693.
13. Srivastava V.K., Prasad D. 2013. DWT-based feature extraction from ECG signal. American Journal of Engineering Research (AJER), 2, 44–50.
14. Ponnusamy M., Sundararajan M. 2017. Detecting and classifying ECG abnormalities using a multi model methods. In Biomedical Research 2017; Special Issue: S81-S89, pp. 81–89.
15. Stantic D., JoJ. Detecting abnormal ECG signals utilising wavelet transform and standard deviation. In Proceedings of *World Academy of Science, Engineering and Technology*, (No. 71), World Academy of Science, Engineering and Technology (WASET), pp. 208–214.
16. Haque A.K.M.F., Ali M.H., Kiber M.A., Hasan M.T. 2009. Detection of small variations of ECG features using wavelet. *ARPN Journal of Engineering and Applied Sciences*, 4, pp. 27–30.
17. Gacek A. 2012. An introduction to ECG signal processing and analysis. In *ECG Signal Processing, Classification and Interpretation*. Springer., London, pp. 21–46.
18. Bendani D., Berrached N.E. 2017. Detection of cardiac arrhythmia by using time domain technique on heart rate variability signals. In 2nd International Conference on Bio-engineering for Smart Technologies (BioSMART). IEEE, pp. 1–4.

19. Lopez A.D., Joseph L.A. 2013. Classification of arrhythmias using statistical features in the wavelet transform domain. In International Conference on Advanced Computing and Communication Systems. IEEE, pp. 1–6.
20. Karthika J.S., Thomas J.M., Kizhakkethottam J.J. 2015. Detection of life-threatening arrhythmias using temporal, spectral and wavelet features. In International Conference on Computational Intelligence and Computing Research (ICCIC). IEEE, pp. 1–4.
21. Celin S., Vasanth K. 2017. Survey on the methods for detecting arrhythmias using heart rate signals. In Journal of Pharmaceutical Sciences and Research Vol 9, Iss. 2, pp. 183–189.
22. Devika M.G., Gopakumar C., Aneesh R.P., Nayar G.R. 2016. *Myocardial infarction detection using hybrid BSS method*. IEEE, pp. 167–172.
23. Limaye H., Deshmukh V.V. 2016. ECG noise sources and various noise removal techniques: A survey. *International Journal of Application or Innovation in Engineering and Management*, 5, 86–92.
24. Guyon I., Gunn S., Nikravesh M., Zadeh L.A. 2008. *Feature Extraction: Foundations and Applications*. Vol. 207, Springer.
25. Sahu M.M., Saxena A., Manoria M. 2015. Application of feature extraction technique: A review. *IJCSIT*, 4, pp. 3014–3016.
26. Guyon I., Elisseeff A. 2006. An introduction to feature extraction. In Guyon I., Nikravesh M., Gunn S., Zadeh L.A. (eds), Feature Extraction. Studies in Fuzziness and Soft Computing, vol 207, Springer: Berlin, Heidelberg, pp. 1–25.
27. Park H. 2013. An introduction to logistic regression: From basic concepts to interpretation with particular attention to nursing domain. *Journal of Korean Academy of Nursing*, 43(2), pp. 154–164.
28. Han J., Pei J., Kamber M. 2014. *Data mining: Concepts and techniques*. In 2011 *on Security, Pattern Analysis, and Cybernetics*. Elsevier, pp. 324–328.

5

Computer Vision for Brain Tissue Segmentation

M. Sucharitha, Chinmay Chakraborty, S. Srinivasa Rao and V. Siva Kumar Reddy

CONTENTS

5.1 Introduction

Magnetic resonance imaging is a frequent technique for clinical examination of brain illnesses (Dolz et al., 2016). Due to the presence of distinct tissues such as grey matter, white matter and cerebrospinal fluid, the shape of the human brain is complex (Thirumurugan et al., 2018). These tissues are important for humans which play a key role in memory, cognition, awareness, and language. However, blurry boundaries make vital tissues such as cerebrospinal fluid, gray matter and white matter difficult to differentiate. Hence, it is difficult for physicians to analyze and differentiate tissues one by one and to become aware of the location of the disease. Computer-aided analysis enhances the efficiency of segmenting gray matter, cerebrospinal fluid and white matter. In the medical analysis of magnetic resonance (MR) images, image segmentation is frequently a preliminary and integral stage. Segmentation algorithms primarily based on regional, texture and histogram thresholds (Bezdek et al., 1993, Jiang and Yang, 2003) are simple; however, good accuracy is not achieved. The threshold is effective and it is easy to section images, but it has some limitations. Firstly, if the threshold is used to locate tissues, it may additionally fail to separate all components due to the fact that the greyscale of the tissues is not in a particular range. Secondly, the spatial properties of an image are not considered. When the cranium is round in shape and covers different tissues, then the place of tissues can be decided and accuracy is improved. As a result of the early-stage sequential image process, the threshold determination is used. Later, Fuzzy C-Means (FCM) (Krinidis and Chatzis, 2010, Hathaway and Bezdek, 2000) and machine learning are introduced. The accuracy is more for clinical image segmentation with the usage of automated segmentation algorithms than for manual calculations. A significant unsupervised clustering approach is the FCM algorithm. The spatial statistics are not taken into account and are not suitable for clustering a noisy image. By incorporating the local spatial information and the gray level information, a new approach for image clustering has been proposed. This is the Reformulated Fuzzy Local Information C-Means (RFLICM) clustering algorithm, in which the information about the spatial context is included in a fuzzy way. The spatial distance is changed by using a local coefficient of variation to limit the noise. In this chapter, automated segmentation and classification of tissues are proposed.

The atlas-based approach is used for intelligence image segmentation and has a complete system framework (Han and Fischl, 2007). Spatial and intensity aspects (Moeskops et al., 2016) are prevented using convolutional neural networks (CNNs). The convolutional neural network proposed by LeCun et al. (1998) is a deep learning approach and has been applied in many fields because it has been an incredible success in image recognition, speech recognition and so on. CNNs attain the convolution weight via the capacity of cyclic convolution and samples with a supervised training mode. The final realization is extracted from unique input and is conducive to classification features. The elements in image recognition are texture, shape and structure. In this chapter, clustering by way of the fuzzy method and CNN for segmenting the brain into three tissue areas are dealt with in detail.

5.2 Materials and Methods

5.2.1 Magnetic Resonance Imaging (MRI)

The kind of image received for brain tissue segmentation is from Magnetic Resonance Imaging, and this section discusses in detail the MRI image acquisition from the OASIS database with a sample image.

MRI is a superior approach utilized for clinical imaging as well as treatment. Magnetic Resonance Imaging (MRI) high-resolution images are used to take a look at human brain improvement and to discover abnormalities. It is a beneficial tool to understand various states of the human brain. MRI shows facts about smooth tissues in the body and it scores well compared to other diagnostic imaging strategies. Scientists from assorted disciplines made it a real-time imaging tool for the brain, heart, lungs and other organs. Its advantages over different diagnostic modalities are its excessive spatial resolution and excellent soft tissue discrimination (Kekre et al., 2011). The advent of an MRI image scan has paved a way for the introduction of many mechanized and computer-supported technologies specifically for clinical image analyses. MRI is receptive to brain atrophy. Structural MRIs and Diffusion Tensor Imaging (DTI) transmit insights into the human intelligence structure. MRIs are used to identify Alzheimer's disease (AD) at a premature state before the occurrence of irreparable damage (Desai and Parmar, 2012).

Recent research on image analysis algorithms has shown that structural MRI tools can instantly divide the brain into anatomic areas and can quantify tissue atrophy in these areas. The Open Access Series of Imaging Studies (OASIS) database was supposed to ensure the availability of brain MRI data sets to scientists. A free MRI data set is facilitated in basic/clinical neuroscience (Marcus et al., 2007).

The following figure indicates the sample of brain image collected from the OASIS database which is processed and segmented for classifying into specific tissues.

5.2.2 Segmentation Methods for Brain Images

In the image processing steps for the classification of medical images, segmentation is the initial and necessary step (Roy and Bandyopadhyay, 2012). Image segmentation is the most well-known way to sort the pixels of an image precisely. It is the procedure of dividing an image into a variety of areas so that every vicinity is homogenous. The segmentation algorithms are typically grounded in two indispensable features of intensity values: discontinuity and similarity (Vokurka et al., 2001). In the first, the technique is to conduct segmentation depending on disconnected shifts in intensity, and the second, segmenting the image into areas that are comparable to predetermined criteria. Medical image segmentation is the main challenge for detecting and locating tumors, diagnostic functions and so on (Rajapakse and Kruggel, 1998).

Image segmentation methods can also be categorized by relying on the Hierarchical Self-Organizing Map (HSOM) (Wells et al., 1996), and feature vector clustering. Vector quantization is the method of partitioning an n-dimensional vector space into M areas to optimize a criterion characteristic when all the points in each area are approximated, utilizing the representation vector Xi associated with that vicinity (Kapur et al., 1998).

Medical images play a fundamental role in healthcare for the diagnosis and treatment of patients. Normally radiologists evaluate medical images primarily based on visual interpretation. However, depending on the experience of the radiologist, analysis is time-consuming and commonly subjective. To overcome this limitation, a computer-aided diagnostic system will become necessary. Artificial intelligence strategies combined with other techniques produce better results than the manual method. In this chapter, the goal is routinely extracting information from an image by way of image segmentation for classifying the tissues.

A lot of research work has been carried out with several methods for image segmentation. An overview of the associated research work performed on image segmentation is introduced in this section. Image analysis is an important task in image segmentation. At the present time, image segmentation has been appreciably applied in the clinical field for diagnosing illnesses, and additionally in a range of applications including object detection, pattern recognition and clinical imaging (Kim et al., 2005). The segmentation of anatomic shapes in the brain performs a fundamental function in neuroimaging analysis. Successful numerical algorithms can assist researchers, doctors and neurosurgeons to check out and diagnose the shape and features of the brain in both health and disease. This has encouraged the need for segmentation methods that are robust in utility involving a vast range of anatomic structure, disorder and image type (Dao and Song, 2004). The mission of image segmentation is the partition of an image into exclusive meaningful areas with homogeneous characteristics. Recently, numerous methods have been developed for segmenting an image using discontinuities or similarities of pixel value, color and the texture of the image (Dong and Xie, 2005). Despite much effort and incredible outcomes in the medical imaging domain, precise segmentation and characterization of anomalies remain a difficult undertaking due to the diverse differences in potential shapes, locations and intensities. Some of the MR image segmentation methods are described as follows.

Thresholds: These can be implemented on an image to determine areas with different intensities, and therefore differentiate between tissue areas represented within the image. But, in images where intensity non-uniformity and noise exist, it may be tough to discover extra thresholds to segment the image without serious misclassification. The application of thresholds is extraordinarily easy, and they continue to be used with the aid of additional processing steps (Aggarwal and Agrawal, 2012).

Region Growing: Regions with homogeneous points are segmented by way of seeding a location in the image.

Rule-Based Segmentation: This is an unsupervised image segmentation where image primitives are inferred and then comprehended through a set of rules.

Atlas-Based Segmentation Method: This approach allows for spatial prior chances and estimates the parameters responsible for initial intensity distribution in an image (Ahmed and Mohamad, 2011).

Edge Detection Techniques: Edges are created at the boundary of areas where there is a sudden change in gray level intensity value. The most popular edge detection techniques are Laplacian of Gaussian (LoG), Sobel, Roberts and Canny operators.

Deformable Models: This is an iterative, model-based technique for the detection of region boundaries by way of utilizing closed parametric curves.

Watershed: This is a gradient-based segmentation technique where different gradient values are regarded as specific heights (Bandhyopadhyay and Paul, 2012).

K-Means Clustering: Also referred to as hard clustering, it is efficaciously employed in various domains like image segmentation, pattern recognition and classifier designs. This approach groups images into *c* classes using data points. The algorithm arbitrarily picks *k* points and each point is assigned to clusters that are closest to its center. Cluster center c_j is revised by calculating its mean, and each cluster is repeated until the system converges. After some finite number of iterations, the algorithm can be demonstrated to converge. The minimization of the objective function is given as in Equation (5.1) (Javed et al., 2014, Chakraborty et al., 2016).

$$J = \sum_{j=1}^{k} \sum_{i=1}^{m} ||x_i^{(j)} - c_j||^2 \quad (5.1)$$

Several segmentation strategies were mentioned and amongst them, the clustering method of image segmentation is preferred. This chapter follows this preference by presenting clustering-based segmentation.

5.2.3 Clustering Techniques

Clustering is an unsupervised technique that divides given statistics into exclusive clusters based totally on their distances (similarity) from each other.

The two primary clustering techniques are

i. Hard clustering
ii. Fuzzy clustering or soft clustering

Each one has its particular characteristics. Normally each point of data is classified into a single cluster in hard clustering methods. But hard segmentation faces many drawbacks such as noise, low spatial resolution, low contrast and intensity inhomogeneity variations.

The overall performance of fuzzy clustering as an image segmentation technique is better compared to the hard clustering method because it retains more information from the unique image.

Among fuzzy clustering methods, more precedence is given to the Fuzzy C-Means (FCM) algorithm. In the fields of clinical imaging, geology and fingerprint recognition, this unsupervised method has been efficiently utilized for analyzing images, clustering and classifier design. Segmentation through fuzzy pixel classification can be acquired using this approach, as FCM tends to classify every pixel into unique classes depending on the ranges of membership. The flexibility in this strategy lets in many applications that these days have been used to process magnetic resonance images. In current times, many new techniques have evolved to improve the FCM algorithm. The objective function of conventional FCM is modified by using it together with the spatial parameter on membership functions.

The spatial term helps to estimate spatially smooth membership functions and also undergoes a more iterative process which is the same as the original FCM. Geometrically Guided FCM (GG-FCM) was proposed, via Noordam et al. (2000), in which a geometrical condition is utilized by way of thinking about the local neighborhood of every pixel. Ahmed et al., in 2002, proposed FCM_S, in which the goal characteristic of conventional FCM is modified to overcome the intensity inhomogeneity. The labeling of a pixel in FCM_S depends on the labels of its immediate neighborhood. Neighborhood labeling is computed in each iteration step, so the procedure is lengthy and time-consuming, which is the main drawback of FCM_S.

Fast Generalized FCM (FGFCM) is developed by including the spatial information which forms a weighted sum image from original images and its neighborhood. FGFCM segmented image is more suitable and also computational time is very small, because clustering depends on the foundation of the gray level histogram.

In the Enhanced FCM algorithm (EnFCM), as well as in FGFCM, an indispensable parameter a (or λ) is used to manage the trade-off between the mean or median filtered image and its corresponding original image. The choice of this parameter is carried out through the use of trial-and-error technique and is normally challenging, considering that it has to preserve a balance between robustness to noise and effectiveness of keeping the details. The inclusion of a novel fuzzy factor into the goal characteristic of the conventional clustering approach enhances the performance and is free of any adjustable parameter.

5.2.4 Fuzzy Clustering Method for Brain Image Segmentation

This article affords brain image segmentation into one-of-a-kind areas such as GM, WM and CSF with the use of conventional Fuzzy C-Means. The conventional fuzzy clustering approach is modified, and methods such as Fuzzy Local Information C-Means (FLICM) and Reformulated Fuzzy Local Information C-Means (RFLICM) clustering are additionally mentioned in detail. Experiments are carried out with medical images for investigating the overall performance of the proposed RFLICM method via segmenting the brain image into different tissue types.

5.2.4.1 Fuzzy C-Means Clustering (FCM)

FCM is usually employed in quite a number of areas, like pattern recognition, analysis of images, segmentation, etc. In the FCM clustering method, a membership degree is allotted to every information factor belonging to a unique class, and the assignment must be in the right cluster. With the help of a smaller membership degree, a data point that lies on the boundary of a cluster may also be assigned to a nearer cluster. The principal goal of the FCM algorithm is then the minimization of objective characteristics. The minimized objective function is proven in Equation (5.2) (Soesanti et al., 2011, Chakraborty, 2019).

$$W_m = \sum_{j=1}^{n}\sum_{i=1}^{c} U_{ij}^{m} \mid\mid x_j - c_i \mid\mid^2 \quad 1 \le m \le \infty \tag{5.2}$$

Using the FCM algorithm, MR images are segmented into three clusters, namely, white matter, gray matter and CSF, relying on cluster facilities and the membership values of each pixel. Thus, using the traditional FCM algorithm, a clustered image is achieved which depends on the number of clusters used. But the drawback of this algorithm is more sensitive to noise, seeing that the spatial information is not considered.

5.2.4.2 Fuzzy Local Information C-Means (FLICM)

The Fuzzy Local Information C-Means clustering (FLICM) algorithm overcomes the drawback of parameter selection in FCM and stimulates the performance of image segmentation. Some characteristics of FLICM are that it is independent of any sort of noise and is free of any parameter selection and also integrates neighborhood spatial and neighborhood gray level concurrently in a fuzzy way. It will automatically resolve neighborhood constraints. The performance of clustering is more advantageous through image details and noise which are finished mechanically utilizing fuzzy local constraints. FLICM uses an original image with the aim of fending off the pre-processing steps which ought to avoid the missing out of image details.

FLICM characteristic makes use of the local similarity measure in a fuzzy way by necessitating noise insensitivity, and also preserves image details. A new factor G_{ki} brought into FLICM's objective function enhances the clustering. The fuzzy component expressed in Equation (5.3) is

$$G_{ki} = \sum_{j \in N_i} \frac{1}{d_{ij}+1}\left(1-u_{kj}\right)^m \left\|x_j - v_k\right\|^2 \tag{5.3}$$

where the neighborhood window center is at the ith pixel, neighboring pixels falling into window around the ith pixel is the jth pixel and the Euclidean distance between pixels i and j is d_{ij}, v_k is the center of the cluster k prototype and u_{kj} is the gray value j related to the kth cluster.

The factor G_{ki} controls a trade-off between image details and noise and is formulated as an artificial parameter. Pixels that influence a local window G_{ki} are flexibly exerted by way of the usage of Euclidean distance from the central pixel. So, G_{ki} reflects the spatial distances from the central pixel. An artificial parameter in FCM_S and FGFCM is tough in contrast to FLICM with spatial distances from the central pixel. Applying fuzzy factor G_{ki}, no-noisy pixels and noisy pixels corresponding to membership values fall in a neighborhood window and converge to a value that balances the pixel's values in the window. Hence FLICM is strong to outliers with its characteristics, together with noise immunity, image details upkeep besides artificial parameters and direct applicability to the authentic image.

FLICM objective function using G_{ki} is defined as in Equation (5.4):

$$J_m = \sum_{i=1}^{N} \sum_{k=1}^{c} \left[u_{ki}^{m} \left\| x_i - v_k \right\|^2 + G_{ki} \right] \tag{5.4}$$

where v_k represents the kth cluster prototype value and u_{kj} represents fuzzy membership of the ith pixel regarding cluster k, N is the data object number and c is the number of clusters. $\left\| x_i - v_k \right\|^2$ is the Euclidean distance between the cluster center v_k and object x_i.

Also, the centers of the cluster and membership partition matrix are carried out as in Equation (5.5):

$$u_{ki} = \frac{1}{\sum_{j=1}^{c} \left(\frac{\left\| x_i - v_k \right\|^2 + G_{ki}}{\left\| x_i - v_j \right\|^2 + G_{ji}} \right)^{1/(m-1)}}$$
$$v_k = \frac{\sum_{i=1}^{N} u_{ki}^{m} x_i}{\sum_{i=1}^{N} u_{ki}^{m}} \tag{5.5}$$

where the initial membership partition matrix is computed randomly.

The objective function is routinely determined even in the absence of prior noise knowledge, which is the main advantage of the FLICM algorithm. Thus, FLICM enhances the clustering performance and for this reason, better segmentation of the brain image into different tissues can be achieved.

5.2.4.3 Reformulated Fuzzy Information C-Means (RFLICM)

The novel method Reformulated Fuzzy Local Information C-Means clustering algorithm (RFLICM) has been advised for brain segmentation. In FLICM, the gray level information and the spatial information included in the fuzzy factor are represented through gray level differences and spatial distances respectively. Spatial information changes depending on the spatial distances from the central pixel. Using spatial distances from the central pixel, the damping extent of neighbors is determined. When the neighborhood pixel has an equal gray level value, the spatial distance is higher, therefore the damping extent is smaller and vice versa.

But in some cases, calculating the damping extent of the neighbors using the spatial distance alone is not efficient. To overcome this conflict, the spatial distance is changed with the aid of the local coefficient of variation. The local coefficient of variation is described in Equation (5.6).

$$C_{u=} \frac{\mathrm{Var}(x)}{(\bar{x})^2} \tag{5.6}$$

where var(x) and $\bar{x}$ denote the variant in pixel values and the mean of particular masks of the image. Using the local coefficient of variation, the damping extent of neighbors is measured based ~~completely~~ on the region of neighboring pixels. When both the neighbor pixel and ~~the~~ central pixel are in identical regions, the neighborhood coefficient of variation relies ~~upon~~ on the gray level difference between them. Computation of the local coefficient of a variant of every pixel is gone through with appreciation to the local window and extra nearby context information is exploited. Hence, modifying the fuzzy factor of FLICM and the new fuzzy factor G_{ki} in terms of C_u is described as follows.

$$G'_{ki} = \begin{cases} \sum_{j \in N_i} \frac{1}{2 + \min\left(\left(C_u^j / C_u\right)^2, \left(C_u / C_u^j\right)^2\right)} \left(1 - u_{kj}\right)^m \\ \qquad \left\| x_j - v_k \right\|^2, \text{if } C_u^j \geq \overline{C_u} \\ \sum_{j \in N_i} \frac{1}{2 - \min\left(\left(C_u^j / C_u\right)^2, \left(C_u / C_u^j\right)^2\right)} \left(1 - u_{kj}\right)^m \\ \qquad \left\| x_j - v_k \right\|^2, \text{if } C_u^j \geq \overline{C_u} \end{cases} \tag{5.7}$$

where C_u and C_u^j symbolize the neighborhood coefficient of variant corresponding to the central pixel and neighboring pixels, ~~and~~ $\bar{C}_u$ is considered as the mean value of C_u^j which is under the nearby window. By the usage of the definition of $\bar{x}$ the objective function of RFLICM can be represented as

$$J_m = \sum_{i=1}^{N} \sum_{k=1}^{c} u_{ki}^m x_i - v_k{}^2 + G'_{ki} \tag{5.8}$$

where v_k represents the kth cluster prototype value, and u_{ki} represents the fuzzy membership of the ith pixel with respect to cluster k, N is the number of the data items and c is the range of clusters. The Euclidean distance between the object x_i and the cluster center v_k is $\left\| x_i - v_k \right\|^2$.

By the usage of the Reformulated Fuzzy Local Information C-Means (RFLICM) algorithm, the segmented output is obtained from the original image.

5.2.5 Convolution Neural Network

Healthcare providers capture huge amounts of data containing valuable signals and information. Because of shape and size variations of anatomy between persons, the automated segmentation of medical images is challenging. Automated segmentation is difficult due to the low contrast of surrounding tissues. The objective is that when input is given, a mathematical model will be created and trained to obtain useful outputs. A mathematical model can learn from data and perform proper predictions from the generalized as well as new data. The generalization ability of the models is generally estimated based on the training of the data. The final model is tested using the test data, after undergoing several iterations of training. Performance is analyzed based on how the model will be simulated when new data is given.

Recent advances in the healthcare field are mainly due to the application of deep learning-based methods. This method can learn the features directly from the imaging data. It is used to separate homogeneous areas for further diagnosis and a treatment pipeline. Deep learning-based image segmentation is hence used as a robust tool in image segmentation. In this chapter, the Convolutional Neural Network (CNN) is used for accurate brain tissue segmentation and is a supervised learning approach method. Mohammad et al., in 2017 proposed CNN, which uses both local features and global contextual features simultaneously. A deep network is a form of computation in which each layer does some computation and stores its output in memory for the next layer to use. CNNs are widely used for image recognition and segmentation. Image features are extracted before operating using a back-propagation neural network (BPN), but CNN itself extracts the useful and necessary features required for performing segmentation. A CNN's basic structure consists of two layers. The extraction of the local features is done by connecting the input of each neuron to the previous layer. The positional relationship between other neurons is determined after extracting the local feature. Another layer is the feature mapping network layer, and each computing layer is composed of multiple feature maps. A feature map is a flat plane in which all neuron weights are equal. The feature mapping structure uses the sigmoid function (Liu et al., 2015) as the activation function of the convolution network. Each convolutional layer in a CNN closely follows a computing layer for local average and second extraction.

A CNN consists of several convolutional layers, pooling layers and fully connected layers followed by one classification layer. When an image is given as input to the CNN, feature maps are obtained by convolving the image with filters. Two to five pooling layers are used to undergo sub-sampling for each map with mean or max-pooling layers. The number of fully connected layers is present after the convolutional layers.

5.3 Experimental Outcomes

The goal is to segment brain MR images (Wright, 1998) into three regions corresponding to GM, WM and CSF. In numerical experiments, the number of clusters chosen to be c=3, corresponding to three tissues. The algorithm is tested on the original images corrupted by salt and pepper and Gaussian noise.

Figure 5.1 shows the original input image (MR1 and MR2) and the image affected with salt and pepper and Gaussian noise of 9%. Clustering results achieved by the conventional FCM algorithm contains a lot of spots. This is because the FCM algorithm fails to incorporate the spatial relationship between neighboring pixels. In FLICM, after incorporating local spatial information, the segmented output is robust to outliers, but some noise remained in the clustered result.

Since segmentation plays a very important role in the classification of normal and abnormal brain tissues, it is noted that compared to the conventional Fuzzy Clustering technique, the novel segmentation RFLICM technique segments the brain tissue more accurately by including spatial and gray level information.

Figure 5.2 shows the output of the MR image obtained by implementing the RFLICM technique which indicates tissues as gray matter, white matter and cerebrospinal fluid (CSF). Better classification of three tissue regions is achieved, since RFLICM eliminates the effect of noise greatly.

Table 5.1 shows the segmentation accuracy of different algorithms on original images added by salt and pepper and Gaussian noise with different noise levels as 9% and 20%. It is observed that the SA value of RFLICM is better than the other two algorithms with different noise levels. The important parameter to determine the accuracy of the proposed algorithm is Segmentation Accuracy (SA). Denoising the performance of three algorithms was compared concerning optimal segmentation accuracy. The sum of correctly classified pixels divided by the sum of the total number of pixels indicates segmentation accuracy.

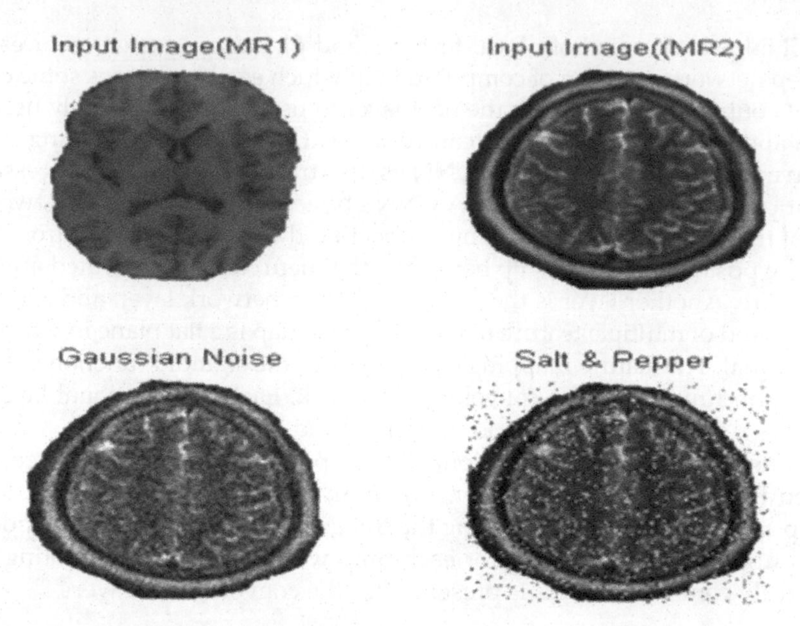

FIGURE 5.1
Input image and noise added image.

$$S = \sum_{i=1}^{c} \frac{A_i \cap C_i}{\sum_{j=1}^{c} C_j} \tag{5.9}$$

where pixels belonging to ith class are A_i and pixels belonging to the same class in the reference segmented image are C_i. The better accuracy obtained for RFLICM is 99.86% for image added with 9% of salt and pepper noise. From the observed outputs and comparisons, it is concluded that the proposed algorithm performance is better than other techniques for segmenting the brain image into different tissues.

The implementation steps are input generation, deep network training and retrieving discovered features. CNN is used for tissue segmentation after extracting the useful features. The structure in this article makes use of two layers as the convolution layer and the pooling layer. After performing the convolution, a couple of feature maps are generated using the convolution layer. By including appropriate weighted values and offset, pixels corresponding to the feature map of each group are modified. In the pooling layer, the sigmoid characteristic is used to get the appropriate function map. Accurate results are obtained with less iteration in contrast to manual and semiautomatic segmentation due to the presence of convolution and pooling layers. The runtime of the system is decreased by way of the use of parallel computing.

5.4 Conclusion

The automatic segmentation of MR brain image is one of the vital issues in clinical imaging. FCM is one of the most well-known clustering approaches and has been widely utilized for medical image segmentation. Even though the conventional FCM algorithm produces

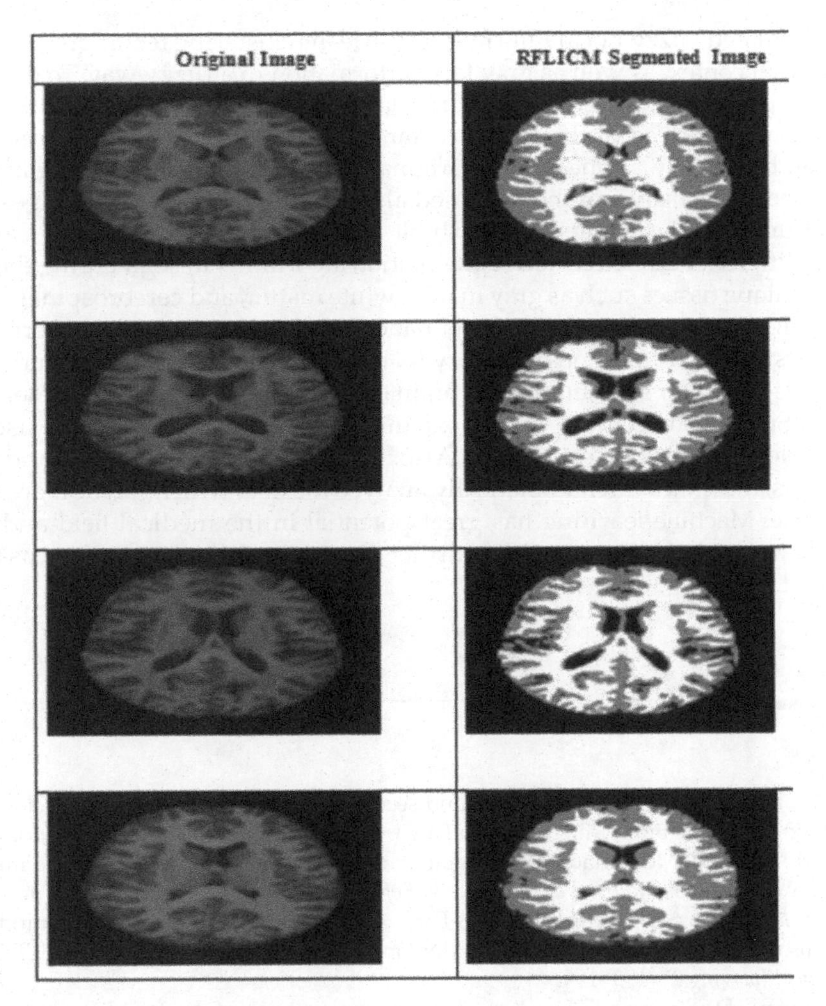

FIGURE 5.2
RFLICM segmented image.

true output for noise-free image segmentation, it fails to segment images corrupted via outliers, noise and other imaging artifacts. We have provided a succinct discussion of our

TABLE 5.1
Segmentation Accuracy

Images	Noise (%)	FCM	FLICM	RFLICM
MR1	Salt & Pepper 9%	97.64	98.24	99.86
	Salt & Pepper 20%	96.56	97.62	98.92
	Gaussian 9%	91.29	98.42	99. 65
	Gaussian 20%	89.57	97.35	98.82
MR2	Salt & Pepper 9%	92.95	98.96	99.54
	Salt & Pepper 20%	90.37	97.52	98.71
	Gaussian 9%	89.29	97.15	99.26
	Gaussian 20%	87.37	95.57	98.89

latest Reformulated Fuzzy Local Information C-Means clustering technique by incorporating local spatial context as well as gray level information in a fuzzy way. To emphasize an automated application, the algorithm is formulated in such a trend via using the local coefficient of variation instead of the spatial distance. The novelty of the proposed technique is that it can be directly applied to the original image without performing any precomputations. The performance of the proposed algorithm is analyzed by doing experiments on medical images. Clustering effects exhibit that the proposed algorithm can function better than different FCM extension segmentation algorithms in segmenting the MR brain image into unique tissues such as gray matter, white matter, and cerebrospinal fluid. In the future, the algorithm, moreover, can be enhanced through introducing a kernel distance measure to its objective function in a fuzzy manner. To conclude, the convolutional neural network is also used for segmenting the brain tissues from MRI and higher segmentation is achieved. Speed and accuracy can be expanded when a deep network is used, since it can extract elements for any set of data. Also, when compared to manual and semiautomatic analysis, machines can automatically analyze the data which can be a great deal and more accurate. Machine learning has great potential in the medical field and this technique can be a criterion of judgment for further diagnosis of diseases as soon as the tissues are identified.

References

Aggarwal, N., and R.K. Agrawal. 2012. First and second order statistics features for classification of magnetic resonance brain images. *Journal of Signal and Information Processing* 3, no. 1: 146–153.

Ahmed, M.M., and D.B. Mohamad. 2011. Segmentation of brain magnetic resonance images MRIs: A review. *International Journal of Advances in Soft Computing & its Applications* 3, no. 3: 18–24.

Ahmed, M.N., Yamany, S.M., Mohamed, N., Fara, A.A., and T. Moriarty. 2002. A modified fuzzy C-means algorithm for bias field estimation and segmentation of MRI data. *IEEE Transactions on Medical Imaging* 21: 193–199.

Bandhyopadhyay, D.S.K., and T.U. Paul. 2012. Segmentation of brain MRI image–A review. *International Journal of Advanced Research in Computer Science and Software Engineering* 2, no. 3, Corpus ID: 7157855.

Bezdek, J.C., Hall, L.O., and L.P. Clarke. 1993. Review of MR image segmentation techniques using pattern recognition. *Medical Physics* 20, no. 4: 1033–1048.

Chakraborty, C. 2019. Computational approach for chronic wound tissue characterization. In *Informatics in Medicine Unlocked*. Elsevier. Vol. 17, pp. 1–10.

Chakraborty, C., Gupta, B., Ghosh, S.K., Das, D., and C. Chakraborty. 2016. Telemedicine supported chronic wound tissue prediction using different classification approach. *Journal of Medical Systems* 40, no. 3: 1–12.

Dao, Z., and C.C. Song. 2004. A novel kernelized fuzzy C-means algorithm with application in medical image segmentation. *Artificial Intelligence in Medicine* 32: 37–50.

Desai, K.D., and S. Parmar. 2012. Effective early detection of Alzheimer's and Dementia disease using Brain MRI Scan Images. *International Journal of Emerging Technology and Advanced Engineering* 2, no.4, 414–417.

Dolz, J., Betrouni, N., and M. Quidet. 2016. Stacking denoising auto-encoders in a deep network to segment the brainstem on MRI in brain cancer patients: A clinical study. *Computerized Medical Imaging and Graphics* 52: 8–18.

Dong, G., and M. Xie. 2005. Colour clustering and learning for image segmentation based on neural networks. *IEEE Transactions on Neural Networks* 16, no. 4: 925–936.

Han, X., and B. Fischl. 2007. Atlas renormalization for improved brain MR image segmentation across scanner platforms. *IEEE Transactions on Medical Imaging* 26: 479–486.

Hathaway, R.J., and J.C. Bezdek. 2000. Generalized fuzzy c-means clustering strategies using Lp norm distance. *IEEE Transactions on Fuzzy Systems* 8: 567–572.

Javed, A., Chai, W.Y., Alenezi, A.R., and N. Kulathuramaiyer. 2014. Enhancement of magnetic resonance images using soft computing based segmentation. *International Journal of Machine Learning and Computing* 41: 73–78.

Jiang, L., and W. Yang. 2003. A modified fuzzy C-means algorithm for segmentation of magnetic resonance images. In *Proceedings VIIth Digital Image Computing: Techniques and Applications.*

Kapur, T., Eric, W., Grimson, L., Kikinis, R., and W.M. Wells. 1998. Enhanced spatial priors for segmentation of magnetic resonance imagery. *Medical Image Computing and Computer-Assisted Intervention*, no. 3: 457–468.

Kekre, D.H., Sarode, D.T., Gharge, S., and M.K. Raut. 2011. Image Segmentation of MRI images using KMCG and KFCG algorithms. In *2nd International Conference and Workshop on Emerging Trends and Technology (ICWET).*

Kim, J., Fisher, J.W., Yezzi, A., Cetin, M., and A.S. Willsky. 2005. A non-parametric statistical method for image segmentation using information theory and curve evolution. *IEEE Transactions on Image Processing* 14, no.10: 1486–1502.

Krinidis, S., and V. Chatzis. 2010. A robust fuzzy local information C-means clustering algorithm. *IEEE Transactions on Image Processing* 19, no.5: 1328–1337.

Lecun, Y., Bottou, L., Bengio, Y., and P. Haffner. 1998. Gradient-based learning applied to document recognition. *Proceedings of the IEEE* 86, no. 11: 2278–2324.

Liu, T., Fang, S., Zhao, Y., Wang, P., and J. Zhang. 2015. Implementation of Training Convolutional Neural Networks, *Computer Vision and Pattern Recognition.*

Marcus, D.S., Wang, T.H., Parker, J., Csernansky, J.G., Morris, J.C., and R.L. Buckner. 2007. Open Access Series of Imaging Studies OASIS: Cross-sectional MRI data in young, middle aged, non-demented, and demented older adults. *Journal of Cognitive Neuroscience* 19, no. 9: 1498–1507.

Moeskops, P., Viergever, M.A., Mendrik, A.M., Vries, L.S., Benders, M.J.N.L., and I. Isgum. 2016. Automatic segmentation of MR brain images with a convolutional neural network. *IEEE Transactions on Medical Imaging* 35, no. 5: 1252–1261.

Mohammad, H., Axel, D., Antoine, B., Aaron, C., Chris, P., and H. Larochelle. 2017. Brain tumor segmentation with deep neural network. In *Medical Image Analysis*. Elsevier, Vol. 5: pp. 18–31.

Noordam, J., Van den Broek, W., and L. Buydens. 2000. Geometrically guided Fuzzy C-means clustering for multivariate image segmentation. *Proceedings of the International Conference on Pattern Recognition* 1: 462–465.

Rajapakse, J.C., and F. Kruggel. 1998. Segmentation of MR images with intensity inhomogeneities. *Image and Vision Computing* 16, no. 3: 165–180.

Roy, S., and S.K. Bandyopadhyay. 2012. Detection and quantification of brain tumor from MRI of brain and its symmetric analysis. *International Journal of Information and Communication Technology Research* 26. Corpus ID: 16450890.

Soesanti, I., Susanto, A., Widodo, T.S., and M. Tjokronagoro. 2011. Optimized fuzzy logic application for MRI brain images segmentation. *International Journal of Computer Science and Information Technology* 5: 137–146.

Thirumurugan, P., Ezhilmathi, N., and P. Shanthakumar. 2018. An automated brain tumour detection and segmentation methods using MRI images–A review. *Journal of Advanced Research in Dynamical & Control Systems* 10: 1678–1681.

Vokurka, E.A., Watson, N.A., Watson, Y., Thacker, N.A., and A. Jackson. 2001. Improved high resolution MR imaging for surface coils using automated intensity non-uniformity correction: Feasibility study in the orbit. *Journal of Magnetic Resonance Imaging* 145: 540–546.

Wells, W.M., Grimson, W.E., Kikinis, R., and F.A. Jolesz. 1996. Adaptive segmentation of MRI data. *IEEE Transactions on Medical Imaging* 15: 429–442.

Wright, G.A. 1998. Magnetic resonance imaging: A review. *IEEE Signal Processing Magazine*, no.2: 56–66.

6

A Study on Energy-Efficient and Green IoT for Healthcare Applications

B. Arthi, M. Aruna and S. Ananda Kumar

CONTENTS

6.1 Introduction

Internet applications have become the order of the day, and have grown rapidly and become inevitable in almost all human activities. This ever-increasing influence of the Internet of Things (IoT) in day-to-day activities gives IoT a pivotal role, resulting in it becoming a key concept in application developments. IoT uses the help of various network devices to transfer and exchange data between physical objects which will be connected to each other. The main task of IoT thus becomes remotely regulating these objects throughout an existing network. While the primary advantage of IoT is to simplify human efforts through logical techniques, it also makes inter-device connections smooth and effective [1]. IoT has become so unique because of its ability to operate with the least amount of human intervention. IoT is a regulated interrelation between the hardware, software, data and services. As the name indicates, things could be any physical device we use in our day-to-day life, ranging from the venetian blind to music systems, air conditioning systems, water/lighting, home theatre, etc. In all these cases, IoT exchanges data between the equipment and the application through Wi-Fi and/or Bluetooth. IoT is prevalent in almost all walks of life and has become an integral part of all sectors of human activity like cities, homes, utilities, city/township development, healthcare, etc. The benefits of IoT are numerous and achieved by means of cost-cutting, effectiveness, efficiency and ease of operation [2]. Like any advancement of science and technology, IoT also has defects and problems when abused. The excessive dependence on IoT combined with the vulnerability of embedded systems and the IT and communication technologies together paves the way for many security threats, piracy and data leaks and causes untold damage to the commercial, political and social fabrics of a country. This chapter is an attempt to deal with those IoT-related risks and security threats and to analyze the major emerging IoT security technology and various research attempts in the field of IoT security [3].

6.1.1 Emerging Technologies, Challenges and Issues in IoT

There is an increased requirement for IoT technologies to coordinate the communication between various devices and the vast user base. The word "things" in IoT indicates the various devices which are equipped with micro-controllers that can transmit and receive information, and the internet means the network facilitating the connection, like Bluetooth or Wi-Fi. This connection is enabled through wireless sensors.

6.1.1.1 Emerging Technologies in IoT

IoT consists of components like RFID readers which initiate transmission of signals and tags. These readers are enabled with actuators, sensors, objects and tags which act as identifiers. These readers help in improving the visibility of products and their location in the retail segment by means of enhanced accuracy, efficiency and quicker processes. These RFIDs also make the process cost-effective by reducing storage space, handling and logistics costs and thereby increase sales by keeping the stock minimal.

6.1.1.1.1 Reprogramming

Sensor nodes are the key element in IoT technologies. The need for reprogramming of these sensors requires the highest attention of the developers. This reprogramming allows changing the functionality of the software in the device during its operation. These devices are implemented at various levels for various applications in different environments. Invariably, these devices, once deployed, become inaccessible.

6.1.1.1.2 *Memory Allocation/De-allocation Techniques in IoTs*

In various IoT applications, devices are required to gather information, analyze and process them and also constantly categorize the data. For these operations, memory space would be required which would, in turn, increase the overall cost of the device [4]. A few applications used in IoT, like hospital applications, require high efficiency of management of data, as any lag of efficiency would cause untold damages to human lives, and therefore during the development of applications in IoT, the requirement of adequate memory and its management plays a vital role. The memory management in conventional OS refers to the methodology of allocating and de-allocating the memory space required for various processes and their threads. The memory management can be assigned in static and dynamic modes. In static mode, the process is simple and efficient for constant memory resources. However, its inability to allocate and de-allocate memory resources to real-time operations makes it a rigid system. In such situations, dynamic memory management can allocate and de-allocate memory resources efficiently during real-time applications.

6.1.1.1.3 *Energy-Efficient Methods for IoT*

With the tremendous growth of IoT and its applications for various sectors, this makes it imperative for IoT to be energy-efficient at all times. In most of the applications, IoT devices are installed in locations which are remote and inaccessible. Therefore, the device needs to consume less energy to be cost-effective. These devices constantly transfer information using the internet, which can consume a sizeable amount of energy. Extensive research is undertaken on energy-efficient protocols and techniques to make future internet use energy-efficient and cost-efficient [5].

6.1.1.1.4 *Intelligent Processing*

Various intelligent computing technologies like cloud computing help IoT in supporting, collecting and managing the information in databases. With the ability of network service providers to process billions of messages instantly through cloud computing, this makes cloud computing the key promoter of IoT.

6.1.1.1.5 *Localization and Context Awareness*

The versatility of IoT applications demands a modern outlook on our perception of localization systems. The context awareness application is of paramount importance in IoT. The influence of location information on the design of existing and future versions of IoT is an ever-growing field of study, and is subject to rigorous research in many ongoing research projects. Therefore, a detailed analysis of the influence of awareness and deployment of localization systems is of utmost importance [6].

6.1.1.2 Challenges and Issues in IoT

Sensing the huge demand for IoT applications in the various gadgets and appliances for day-to-day life, commercial entities in the market are working hard on introducing IoT applications into their products and services and are ready to invest heavily in development of IoT in them [7, 8]. While praising the huge positive impact of IoT in various sectors of life, we cannot ignore the risks and challenges the system entails as well.

6.1.1.2.1 Privacy

Privacy is perhaps the most compromised element in the IoT sector. IoT involves transfer and exchange of personal data between devices, and thus is susceptible to leakage and entails trust and privacy issues. At a certain stage, data privacy becomes the major crisis faced by IoT developers and beneficiaries, as the data generated, shared and used by various connecting devices becomes open to breaches and abuses [9]. Damages on privacy due to extensive use of IoT can be mitigated by bringing into place suitable privacy agreements, non-disclosure agreements, etc. and implementing appropriate technology-based security checks.

6.1.1.2.2 Security

Another equally worrisome area of disadvantage of the explosive growth of IoT is that of security. In today's world of advanced data use and exchange among devices, users and databases, and even sensitive data/information, are accessible to multiple agencies, wherein lies the threat of misuse or abuse of data. It could prove fatal to the life, safety and security of personnel and properties. Cybercrimes could become rampant in an IoT-based society. More and more advanced and effective technologies to overcome these threats are the need of the hour [6].

6.1.1.2.3 Reliable Communication

Strong and reliable communication channels are an inevitable element for the development of IoT. Now with the advent of 5G, transmission of data between devices has become many times faster than 4G. Such interventions like 5G are believed to bring a very high level of performance and scale to cater to the huge client base consisting of millions of mobile users [6, 10]. Both fixed and mobile technologies of IoT are currently prevalent. Cyber-physical systems supported by two-way communication without much loss of data and with the utmost reliability, enable the creation of new services and applications for IoT [11].

6.1.1.2.4 Power Consumption

Adequate attention needs to be paid to developing alternate power sources for the operation of communication nodes in IoT. Resources like mechanical energy need to be evaluated. The devices associated with IoT are deployed in remote locations in many cases. Therefore, development of more energy-efficient devices and harnessing of alternate sources like mechanical energy has become crucial for IoT in the current advancement of IoT [9].

6.1.1.2.5 Bandwidth

Internet is the lifeblood of IoT. The availability of reliable and uninterrupted internet connectivity with good bandwidth is mandatory for proper use of IoT applications [3]. Strong connection or bandwidth of internet is required, as millions of devices based on IoT would operate across the globe at a given point of time, all depending on the internet.

6.1.1.2.6 Interoperability

Interoperability, or in simpler words, adaptability of the application across multiple devices and operating platforms is a key element in the success of IoT [5]. Very often users may be using various gadgets with various platforms and would want the IoT to run across the wide range of products and platforms [12].

6.1.1.2.7 Architecture Challenge

Communications in IoT are through a wireless channel which is automatic, and work in a dynamic manner. The inter-connected devices and sensors, such as CCTV, access control systems using biometric and parallel sensors often communicate from non-accessible, remote locations [5]. Such services are expected to work seamlessly at any given point of time and transfer the relevant information as required for the specific communication, thus making these services independent and mobile.

6.1.1.2.8 Hardware Challenge

Constant research and the development of hardware is a necessity to evolve cost-effective and easy to use devices which are able to inter-connect with other devices for the transfer of communication using Wi-Fi or Bluetooth technologies. The requirements of IoT applications based on the varied needs of different sectors are for smart systems which are intelligent and autonomous in bringing in new services as required [7].

6.1.1.2.9 Technical Challenge

The heterogeneous architectures in the existing networking technologies and applications make IoT technology more complex for varied reasons. IoT caters to different sectors with specific applications relevant to a particular industry use, hence the services required in the IoT vary in the different environments wherein networking technologies also vary [7]. Based on the requirements, the exchange of information happens through varied networks such as cellular, WAN, LAN and RFID technologies.

6.1.2 Application of IoT

6.1.2.1 Applications, Features and Products of IoT

After the phenomenal development of computers and the internet, now IoT has assumed the third position in revolutionizing the technology world. The development of IoT-based applications has made it the emerging innovation in the modern world [13]. The inter-connection of various devices and the internet in IoT results in the flow of huge amounts of data being saved and processed in a smart way. The applications of IoT vary from sector to sector including, but not limited to, personal, healthcare, industrial and national applications. Currently IoT has steadily gained traction in many core sectors and there has been a deployment of IoT applications in various sectors. Such implementation requires hardware, middleware, internet service providers and a user interface. The communication of the various devices which act as services interacting with the environment, the people and inter-connected devices, enable the performance of tasks independently with minimal human interference in a secured and automated environment. The IoT-based applications require the latest technologies along with advanced readers like RFID and UI interface for better visualization, along with adequate storage capacity to store relevant information for the required time period. The current versions of IoT technologies are the result of developing the right architecture which enables optimal energy conservation.

6.1.2.2 Smart Homes

IoT has played a remarkable role in the management of gadgets and appliances in our homes, like safety, security and automation devices, sensors and entertainment gadgets.

The advent of IoT in such household operations has enabled better management of these devices due to its cost-effectiveness, accuracy and ease of operation [2].

6.1.2.3 Wearable Technology

IoT has also made its inevitable presence in wearable gadgets and devices, like smart wrist watches, smart back-packs, etc. These wearable devices make a traveler more independent and prepared all the time. These devices can be seen in use quite commonly in today's world [14].

6.1.2.4 Smart City

Today's cities are being transformed into smart cities with the influence of IoT. IoT has played its role in almost all aspects of city life, making information and facilities available for city dwellers at their convenience. The reach of IoT is so vast in smart cities that it has application in street lights, pedestrian crossings, conveniently identifying parking lots, automated notification for garbage disposal, surveillance systems and spontaneous notification of accidents and automated arrangement of responses from the specific authorities [15]. Effective vehicular traffic flow management is another key area benefitting from the introduction of IoT. Special care is to be taken in development of an OS for smart city applications, keeping in mind the need for real-time notifications, privacy of personal information and less bandwidth consumption requirements.

6.1.2.5 Smart Grid

With the addition of IoT applications to the conventional power grid systems, it has made the transmission system into a smart grid. In a smart grid, the IoT monitors and analyzes the power consumption of the end users, which could be individuals, commercial buildings and factories. These applications gather data from these end users' consumption and analyzes the data with the transmission of power from the source. This enables tracking of various patterns of power consumption and transmission losses [13]. An IoT-enabled power grid also helps in identifying problems areas like short circuits or other possible hardware malfunctions to avoid wastage of power or a complete blackout of the grid system. These applications help the authorities in understanding the usage analytics based on the consumption patterns of the end users and helps them to better manage the grid system [2]. Development of an OS for these applications requires devices using low bandwidth and energy consumption.

6.1.2.6 Smart Industries

The application of the IoT in the industrial segment is primarily focused on improving and optimizing the industrial operation. IoT is used as an effective tool to accelerate growth opportunities for the industries. The growth of the industry can be accelerated by the increase in production using smart technologies and transforming the industrial workforce. For industrial modernization to optimize operations in an industry intelligent devices need to be implemented [16]. Implementation of IoT applications in large enterprises could be challenging in view of designing the right architecture for the applications that can bring in optimal solutions and feasible solutions. Smart grids, robotics and the digital industry are some examples [2]. IoT has revolutionized the methodology of control processing, monitoring of the industrial environment and the product life-cycle, pollution control, etc. The design and development of an OS for these industrial applications necessitate the use of suitable devices with low energy consumption, low bandwidth and high reliability.

6.1.2.7 Smart Traffic

With emerging applications, the driving experience has been enhanced with people being connected with the Things. At the touch of the fingertips, we are able to access the IoT at any given point of time. The integrating of technologies over IoT has helped us in finding the commonalities in managing various applications using the same method. This has helped in bringing changes in customer applications using the technologies in gathering the varied information available. In the field of transportation, IoT is playing a pivotal role in transforming it into smart transportation. It is estimated that by 2020, 75% of the cars in the world will be IoT-based. This transformation will also bring challenges in capturing the real-time data, improvising on-time delivery, improving fuel efficiency and fleet management to improve performance [13]. The objective of IoT is to provide environment friendly green vehicles and intelligent transportation. An emerging application is smart taxis, which are driverless. With the possibility of knowing the temperature, fuel and oil levels of the vehicle through cloud-based applications, the end user will be able to access all the information pertaining to the vehicle at any point in time using their mobile devices. Intelligent traffic guidance, along with intelligent vehicle control, will revolutionize the smart transportation sector. A few of the challenges in the sector would be real-time scheduling, security, remote monitoring and the road coordination program. These gaps need to be addressed by developing the right software applications [17].

6.1.2.8 Smart Healthcare

Healthcare plays an integral role in the well-being of humans. Whether it be hospitals, nursing homes or dentistry, it focuses on treating the ailments of people across all age groups. With growing technology, we are noticing advances in the treatments using the latest technology [18]. These have led to innovations in new technology-oriented treatments and bringing in smart healthcare solutions. This solution helps in managing the information about the patients in an error-free manner. In healthcare, the smart application needs to be based on real-time information processing without any margin of error. The application developers focusing on the domain needs ensure that real-time data processing happens in a secure environment with security features and also with lesser bandwidth for the information processing. In the medical field, smart solutions are not only focused on bringing intelligent solutions for the treatment of the ailments, but are also looking at improving the operational efficiency of the hospital management, patient monitoring and personnel monitoring. The smart applications had enabled the hospitals to reach out to the remote location where such treatments were not possible in earlier days.

6.1.2.9 Smart Retail

IOT has revolutionized the retail industry with its innovative applications. IoT-based solutions are enabling sales along with making the industry into a smart retail industry. The applications provide information on customer behavior and the analysis of this is improving sales [1]. These applications also focus on improving store efficiency and quality requirements based on customer needs. The applications also provide analytics on the number of people entering the outlets on a monthly, weekly and hourly basis on a regular day and on weekends. IoT has enabled the retail industry to have smart retail solutions for the supermarkets and the hypermarkets. One such application would be a smart self-management system in a retail outlet. A few applications are used as marketing strategies in the retail stores, such as smart signage boards [19]. The consumption of the batteries by the OS and the bandwidth for information gathering and transfer will be a major concern for these applications.

6.1.2.10 Smart Supply Chain

IoT-based smart solutions for supply chain functions have been developed that provide solutions for complex structures in the supply chain function. Organizations have internal and external stakeholders based out of different location globally, and the application acts as a single platform for the information of all the stakeholders viz. customers, sales department, production facility and the logistic department. The application assists stakeholders at each level of the trade starting with the customer by helping him in placing an e-order. The product can be tracked until delivery using a unique tracking ID. One of the IoT-based applications is a product enabled with an RFID [20]. The RFID holds all the information about the product and it can be tracked on a real-time basis till the delivery point. All the information about the product in the supply chain cycle is accessible to the customer and the supplier through a mobile application as well. The main advantages are accuracy of transactions, quality and quantity, speed of delivery and cost savings.

6.1.2.11 Smart Agricultural

The ever-changing global climate poses a serious threat to food resources, among many other threats caused by global warming. The brunt of this climate change is borne by almost all beneficiaries of natural resources, like farmers and fishermen and the like [21]. Interventions based on IoT are a boon to the agricultural industry, and can and already have started being used in monitoring and analyzing resources like water, soil and climatic conditions. With IoT-based solutions, a sustainable approach in the field of agricultural production has become possible. The smart applications enable increasing productivity, along with tracking the entire supply chain of the produce till it reaches the end users. Optimization of energy efficiency should be the focus of the OS developers while identifying innovative solutions in this sector.

6.2 Green Internet of Things

A green campus can be built to save energy using Internet of Things in which Green IoT is the practice of design, manufacture, usage and disposal of computers and related components without affecting the environment.

IoT plays a vital role in terms of aiding livelihoods, healthcare, agriculture monitoring and, in the near future, transportation. Green IoT [22] enables an eco-friendly environment by making use of facilities and storages that help in preserving natural wealth and human health.

- Green design facilitates designing energy-efficient green IoT-related computer systems and cooling maintenance of its components
- Green fabrication produces computers systems and other related components without affecting our environment
- Green consumption enables us to minimize power consumption of computers
- Green disposal helps in restoring or reutilizing old systems and also recycling the unwanted components

Green computing focuses on the following areas and activities,

- A design for environmental sustainability and its risk mitigation
- Energy-efficient computing, its power management and usage of renewable energy sources
- Data centers design, layout and location, server virtualization
- Responsible recycling and disposal
- Regulatory compliance, assessment tools and methodology, and green metrics and eco-labeling of its products

The following are the principles to achieve Green IoT and to reduce carbon emission [23].

- The size of the network should be reduced using efficient routing algorithms in order to achieve better energy savings
- Efficient sensing techniques should be used in order to save a lot of energy by collecting only required data
- Adopt hybrid architecture in order to condense energy consumption
- Create efficient policies to reduce energy consumption since it has a direct impact
- Use intelligent trade-offs in order to save energy and reduce costs

6.2.1 Emerging Technologies, Challenges and Issues in Green IoT

The enabling technologies for Green IoT using ICT technologies enable subscribers to gather, store, access and manage information. Therefore, greening ICT technologies [24] play an essential role in Green IoT which provide various benefits to the environment by decreasing the energy used for designing, manufacturing and distributing ICT-enabled devices and equipment [25]. Greening ICT enables technologies for Green IoT [26] which include the following techniques (Table 6.1).

6.2.2 Applications of Green IoT

IoT has made noteworthy changes in our environment wherein Green IoT will make extensive changes to our future life and our day-to-day activities with a lot of wearable devices, sensors and drone technology that can work and interact with each other intelligently to carry out all the tasks in making our environment green [27]. Therefore, Green IoT applications should strive towards the reduction of carbon emissions, energy-saving, minimizing hazardous pollution from IoT and creating an eco-friendly environment.

TABLE 6.1

Green ICT: Emerging Techniques Adopted in Green IoT

S.No.	Green RFID	Green WSN	Green CC	Green M2M	Green DC	Green CN	Green Internet
1	Green RFID is a wireless communication system Automated data collection	Green Wireless Sensor Network is a wireless communication and sensing periodic data collection and notification sensor	Green Cloud Computing [9] provides unlimited computation, storage and service over the internet	Intelligent machine to machine (M2M) communication. Cognitive Radio (CR) technique is a combination of electronic and computer network	Green Data Centers act as a repository for storage, dissemination and management of data	Green Communication Network enables 5G techniques which aims to reduce energy utilization and to provide green communication to make healthy environments	Green internet efficiently reduces power consumption
	To make the world greener by reducing vehicle emissions [28], saving energy and improving waste disposal techniques	To maximize energy efficiency, to widen network lifetime, to reduce relay nodes and to minimize system budget.	To promote eco-friendly products, to reduce hazardous materials usage, to increase energy consumption and to improve old and waste products' recyclability	To make huge numbers of machines communicate and collaborate, to share information, to make decisions intelligently	Renewable or green energy sources are used	To reduce CO2 emissions, less exposure to radiation and improve energy-efficiency	Green internet in WAN, focus on power consumption in data network
	Unmanned Aerial Vehicle (UAV) battery and RFID reader detection range	Sensor nodes – sleep mode to save energy consumption	To design and manufacture devices which consume less energy with minimum resource utilization	Adjust the transmission power	Energy efficient context-aware broker (e-CAB)	Communication between machines and humans with improved reliability and quality of service	
2	Energy-efficient techniques and protocols	Energy depletion – generate power from the environment	Power-saving virtual machine (VM) techniques	Communication protocols designed	Dynamic power-management	Energy efficiency using Next Generation Networks (NGN).	Dynamic topology management method
3	RFID tag size should be reduced	Radio optimization techniques – energy-efficient cognitive radio	Energy-efficient resource allocation mechanisms	Activity-based scheduling	Energy-efficient hardware design	Enhance the capacity and data rate with high QoS	Green internet routing technique are designed to achieve renewable and non-renewable energy

(*Continued*)

TABLE 6.1 (CONTINUED)

Green ICT: Emerging Techniques Adopted in Green IoT

S.No.	Green RFID	Green WSN	Green CC	Green M2M	Green DC	Green CN	Green Internet
4		Data reduction mechanisms	Effective and accurate models and evaluation approaches	Joint energy-saving mechanisms	Energy-aware routing algorithms are used		Energy-efficiency of hand-held devices
5		Energy-efficient routing technique	Energy-saving policies	Energy harvesting in CR	Data centers power model	Stochastic geometry approach	
6	Applications [29] such as transportation, production tracking, regulatory compliance returns, shipping, receiving, inventory control, and recalls management	Applications such as fire detection, object tracking, environmental monitoring, industrial process monitoring, evolving constraints in the military, control of machine health monitoring	Multi-Method Data Delivery (MMDD) for Sensor-Cloud (SC)	CR-based smart meters to remote-area power management (RAPM). Flexible, high-capacity and cost-effective 4G long-term evolution (LTE) technology	DC of air conditioning system includes environmental monitoring, air conditioning, communication, temperature control and ventilation	Applications such as robotics communication, interaction with humans and robotics, e-health, media, transport and logistics, e-learning, e-governance, public safety, automotive and industrial systems, etc.	

6.2.2.1 Smart Green Cities

- *Smart Traffic Management* prevents vehicle emissions that harm the planet due to heavy traffic [28]
- *Smart Parking* directs people to available parking so that it saves time for the people who are caught in traffic jams [29]
- *Smart Water Conservation* monitors water consumption which helps to detect water leaks, evaluate water flow rates and also provide smart city water usage statistics
- *Smart Waste Management System* provides a sustainable environment which controls waste production, mostly by recycling the waste [30]
- *Smart Energy Metering* helps to track the energy used in homes to create proper utility bills and protect the Earth [31]

6.2.2.2 Smart Green Home

- Green IoT facilitates a home with a central remote-controlled computer/smartphone to provide a lighting facility, heating/cooling and electronic devices through voice commands
- It can provide removal of waste, ultrasonic showers, beds that make themselves
- It suggests outfits based on our desires and on weather conditions
- It provides electronic soundproof rooms and regulated sunlight for windows and walls that provide warmth/cooling (Table 6.2).

6.2.2.3 Smart Green Healthcare

At present smart green healthcare attempts to provide patients with green hospitals and green equipment to provide energy-efficient solutions to diagnose disease with ultra-low or zero-energy sources intelligently [32].

TABLE 6.2

Smart Home Technologies

Smart Home Features	Technology Used
Smart lighting	Wink Philips Hue
Smart home preheating using thermostat control mechanisms	Nest
Household essentials	Amazon Dash Button Smart Fridges
Intelligent surveillance	Protect, Vivint, Abode
Smart home security	August
Smart conservation of water usage	Nebia
Smart Wi-Fi coverage blanket	Eero Plume
Intelligent hygiene Air quality	iRobot Braava Airmega

- *Smart remote monitoring* allows doctors or nurse to remotely monitor a patient's heart rate or blood pressure
- *Smart self-management of chronic diseases* like diabetes or high blood pressure, measuring and managing their condition over time
- *Smart performance improvement* allows athletes to monitor their performance and also rehabilitation services
- *Smart behavior adaptation* helps patients on a regular basis to stop smoking, to start exercising, to decrease their stress levels, or to improve their sleeping habits
- *Smart detection and diagnosis* in healthcare data can be used to diagnose a patient and strive to provide them the best treatment
- *Smart healthcare services* provide better patient care quality, enhance access to patient care and reduce their care costs

6.2.2.4 Smart Green Grid

- It improves the efficiency of transmission and distribution of electrical energy, power generation and reduce consumption loss [33]
- It distributes electrical energy whenever required and increases electrical energy based on worldwide demand
- It always ensures the integration of high-quality renewable power generation and distribution
- It offers decentralized power generation so that consumers utilize on-site power
- It provides users a smart way to reduce electricity bills based on the utilization of electronic devices with the least priority
- A smart grid system helps in balancing the load since it is not steady over time and also advises consumers to decrease their power consumption
- It offers affordable management and operational expenses
- A smart grid helps in spotting power theft and power equipment failures

6.2.2.5 Smart Agriculture

- *Smart Labor* appears on farms and performs tasks such as planting and watering, harvesting and sorting in order to produce quality food with much less manpower [32]
- *Intelligent Tractors* include cameras and vision systems, GPS, remote monitoring and advanced techniques for object detection and avoidance
- *Smart Seeding system* includes geo-mapping and sensor data for specifying density, moisture, nutrient levels and quality of soil during the seeding process
- *Smart Watering and Irrigation system* helps in obtaining data from sensors about the fields to carry out irrigation as required
- *Smart Weeding and Pest Control system* include cameras, sensors and sprayers to detect the pests and apply pesticides accordingly [34]
- *Smart Harvesters* involves picking fruit or vegetables and constantly watching fields to identify when trees/plants are ready for harvesting ripened crops

6.3 Energy Efficiency in WBAN for IoT

6.3.1 Introduction

The population level of aged people has increased in all the countries, so healthcare technology has to be increased to take care of these aged people. For example, in a recent development, biosensors are used to monitor the human body and the sensed data are sent to the centralized server for analysis and storage. This system used the Body Area Sensor network where the patient is experiencing mobility issues due to complications from staying in the same place for a long period of time in hospital, and the data is gathered from the mobile patient and transferred to the centralized server which is more advanced than the mobile healthcare framework [35]. As per the survey, cardiovascular disease (CVD) is the cause of 30% of all global deaths, as per the World Health Organization (WHO). There are 17.5 million people who die from heart attacks or strokes every year and this statistic increased to 20 million in 2015. These deaths can be reduced and prevented by using a proper healthcare system. Frequent monitoring and regular treatment will minimize the human loss [36, 37].

A WBAN (Wireless Body Area Network) contains many portable low power autonomous sensor nodes used to monitor the functions of the human body for healthcare. Figure 6.1 shows the pictorial representation of a WBAN structure. Communication takes place between local sensors and remote monitoring devices. The sensors deployed within skin are called in-body sensors, and those outside the body are called on-body sensors. Some of the ongoing and completed projects in WBAN for the benefit of patients and the advancement of medical technology are CodeBlue, Mobihealth, iSIM and UbiMon for healthcare systems. As per the discussion, the patients should be monitored continuously using the WBAN, so that other diseases such as hypertension, Parkinson's disease, renal failure, post-operative monitoring, stress and also the prevention of sudden infant death syndrome can be controlled and monitored. Energy-efficiency is a very important task in WBAN because the sensor nodes are battery-powered devices with only a limited

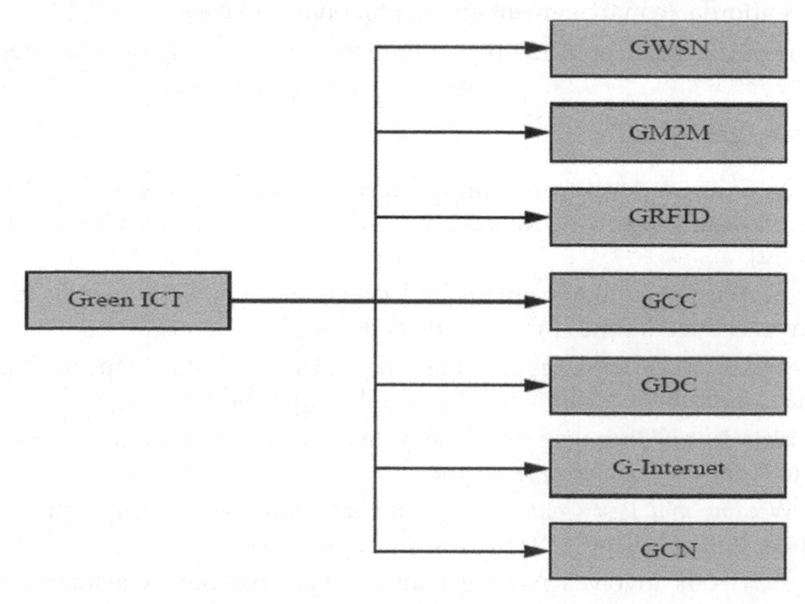

FIGURE 6.1
Green ICT: techniques for Green IoT.

life-span. Sometime the physical characteristics of the nodes may damage human tissue. Though it works on a battery, it directly affects the MAC (Medium Access Control) protocol. So designing an energy-efficient MAC protocol is a major issue for low transmission, low processing power and low cost sensor networks [38–40].

6.3.2 Energy Efficient Protocols

The MAC protocol was developed to increase the lifetime of the network by minimizing power consumption through increasing the sleep mode of the node based on the on-demand wake-up executed by the controller. The wake-up is based on the radio frequency by using the additional circuits and a wake-up table is introduced using a real-time scenario [41]. IEEE 802.15.1 for short-range communication was developed for cable replacement and it will support multi-hop communication and high-energy consumption compared to other MAC protocols [42]. Most of the WBAN is based on the IEEE 802.15.4 MAC standard; this standard is very close and suitable for WBAN applications so it has been adapted for low data rates for a star network [43].

6.3.3 IEEE 802.15.4 Superframe Structure

6.3.3.1 Description of IEEE 802.15.4 MAC Protocol

Most of the work, and our work also, is based on IEEE 802.15.4, so we will describe this standard in detail. It consists of two different access modes which work in star or peer-to-peer networks. With medium access without a beacon interval, it works similarly to the CSMA/CA protocol. The other mode is beacon-enabled with CSMA/CA. The IEEE802.15.4 describes a beacon-enabled superframe structure which is divided into two parts: the active period and the inactive period. Again, the active period is classified into three sections overall, consisting of 16 time slots. The slots are further divided into one slot for the beacon where the centralized node can alert the nodes in the network maximum of seven slots for a Contention Free Period (CFP); the most urgent data are communicated to the coordinator in this slot without any delay. The slot allocation is done by the coordinator. The rest of the slots for the Contention Access Period (CAP) execute the CSMA/CA concept. The duration between the two beacons is called the Beacon Interval (BI).

Where the Beacon Order (BO) decides the length of BI, the MAC Superframe Order (SO) decides the length of the Superframe. The second part of the IEEE802.15.4 is the inactive period, when the nodes will go into the low listening period and will not communicate any data to the central coordinator. A Base Superframe Duration is calculated as a base slot duration with multiple numbers of superframe slots. The base's slot duration by default is 60, and the number of slots is 16 by default. As per the standard defined [43] in the MAC frame format, frame control field and beacon frame are defined in this section.

Octets: 2	**1**	**0/2**	**0/2/8**	**0/2**	**0/2/8**	**Variable**	**2**
Frame control	Sequence number	Destination PAN identifier	Destination address	Source PAN identifier	Source address	Frame payload	FCS
			Addressing Field				
MHR						MAC payload	MFR

IEEE 802.15.4 MAC Frame Format

Bits: 0–2	3	4	5	6	7–9	10–11	12–13	14–15
Fame type	Security enabled	Frame pending	Ack request	Intra PAN	Reserved	Dest Address mode	Reserved	Source Address mode

Frame Control

Octets: 2	1	4/10	2	Variable	Variable	Variable	2
Frame control	Sequence number	Addressing Field	Superframe specification	GTS fields	Pending address fields	Beacon payload	FCS
MHR			MAC payload				MFR

Beacon Frame Format

This protocol use the combination of a contention access period (CAP) for a set of normal and critical data, where different priorities are assigned to a set of nodes based on the traffic, the priority nodes vary the window size and the security features are added to prevent illegal access, and a contention free period (CFP) for huge data works based on TDMA. The superframe consists of a beacon followed by CAP1, and CFP and CAP2 are used to send the remaining priority of CAP1. The contention window size varies due to priority; the higher the priority, the smaller the contention window used [44]. A DQ MAC is proposed, that is, a Distributed Queue MAC protocol, for energy-saving based on the two approaches. If the load is low, it executes the random access process, and if the load is increased gradually, it processes the reservation technique. For that, all the stations in DQ-MQC maintain two queues: one is the collision resolution queue, and the other is the data transmission queue [45]. WBAN is used to monitor the patient's health condition and the mobility of the patient locally and also remotely using the internet [49]. Here the study is compared with the performance of the remote patient monitoring with Zigbee MAC which is based on IEEE 802.12.4 [46]. It developed a new MAC protocol based on IEEE 802.15.4 by introducing the concepts of polling access and emergency transmission in the Contention Access Period in 802.15.4. The transmission is executed for a two-hop in and out body sensor network [47]. A priority is defined for various events and based on that, three priority queues are derived from the priority assigned for different events and different traffic. QoSs parameters are compared by varying queue length and queue delay [48].

It uses a star topology to execute protocol. The centralized node is a PAN coordinator. It may be a sensor1, PDA [50] or any mobile device, which is capable of updating GTS availability to all its associated nodes periodically.

6.4 Conclusion

IoT will be creating a new generation of society enabled with information and knowledge. The application of IoT is unlimited due to advances in technologies and the ease of integrating multiple devices and components, especially in the consumer sector, where most of the home appliances and systems are now integrated with smartphones. These advances have led to the requirements of different technologies to support such integration. The future of IoT depends on having highly portable technologies which can work for different requirements. This has led to the development of technical specifications and the standards which will allow seamless communication between IoT devices and the components. With Wi-Fi, it is now possible for the end users to connect to components anywhere in the world. This will result in the seamless transfer of billions of bytes of data while the devices and the components are communicating with each other. The security of such data will become critical and hence security measures to manage the data and the relevant technologies to secure the data should also emerge alongside. With these data becoming critical, it is important for governments to enable policies and systems to be put in place for private organizations to use it in an ethical manner. The scope for the IoT to grow in the future is exciting, as are the improvements in productivity along with the accuracy of information available to make informed decisions. With these, we can expect great things coming to the world by connecting with IoT.

References

1. Perera C., Chi H. L. Srimal J., and Min C. 2014. A survey on internet of things from industrial market perspective. *IEEE Access* 2, 1660–1679.
2. Lee I., and Kyoochun L. 2015. The Internet of Things (IoT): Applications, investments, and challenges for enterprises. *Business Horizons* 58, no. 4, 431–440.
3. Singh D., Gaurav T., and Antonio J. J. 2014. A survey of Internet-of-Things: Future vision, architecture, challenges and services. In *2014 IEEE World Forum on Internet of Things (WF-IoT)*, Seoul, South Korea 6–8 March, IEEE catalog number: ISBN: CFP1418V-POD 978-1-4799-5071-3, pp. 287–292.
4. Dong W., Chun C., Xue L., and Jiajun B. 2010. Providing OS support for wireless sensor networks: Challenges and approaches. *IEEE Communications Surveys & Tutorials* 12, no. 4, 519–530.
5. Alqassem, I. 2014. Privacy and security requirements framework for the internet of things (IoT). 36th International Conference on Software Engineering, Hyderabad India May, 2014, Association for Computing Machinery New York, United States, pp. 739–741.
6. Xu T., James B. W., and Miodrag P. 2014. Security of IoT systems: Design challenges and opportunities. In *2014 IEEE/ACM International Conference on Computer-Aided Design (ICCAD)*, San Jose California November, 2014, ISBN: 978-1-4799-6277-8, pp. 417–423.
7. Tsai C. W., Chin F. L., and Athanasios V. V. 2014. Future Internet of Things: Open issues and challenges. *Wireless Networks* 20, no. 8, 2201–2217.
8. Gazis V., Manuel G., Marco H., Alessandro L., Kostas M., Alexander W., and Florian Z. 2015. Short paper: IoT: Challenges, projects, architectures. In *2015 18th International Conference on Intelligence in Next Generation Networks*, pp. 145–147.
9. Trequattrini R., Riad S., Alessandra L., and Rosa L. 2016. Risk of an epidemic impact when adopting the internet of things: The role of sector-based resistance. *Business Process Management Journal* 22, no. 2, 403–419.
10. Stankovic J. A. 2014. Research directions for the internet of things. *IEEE Internet of Things Journal* 1, no. 1, 3–9.
11. Polk T., and Turner, S. 2011. Security challenges for the internet of things. In *Workshop on Interconnecting Smart Objects with the Internet, Internet Architecture Board (IAB), Czech Technical University in Prague*.
12. Atzori L., Antonio I. and Giacomo M. 2010. The internet of things: A survey. *Computer Networks* 54, no. 15, 2787–2805.
13. Chen Y. K. 2012. Challenges and opportunities of internet of things. In *17th Asia and South Pacific Design Automation Conference*, ASP-DAC 2012, Jan. 30–Feb. 2, 2012, Sydney, Australia, pp. 383–388. IEEE.

14. Wei J. 2014. How wearables intersect with the cloud and the internet of things: Considerations for the developers of wearables. *IEEE Consumer Electronics Magazine* 3, no. 3, 53–56.
15. Zanella A., Nicola B., Angelo C., Lorenzo V., and Michele Z. 2014. Internet of things for smart cities. *IEEE Internet of Things Journal* 1, no. 1, 22–32.
16. Breivold H. P., and Kristian S. 2015. Internet of things for industrial automation–Challenges and technical solutions. In *2015 IEEE International Conference on Data Science and Data Intensive Systems*, (DSDIS), Sydney, Australia, pp. 532–539. IEEE.
17. Thakur T. T., Ameya N., Sheetal V., and Manjiri G. 2016. Real time traffic management using Internet of Things. In *2016 International Conference on Communication and Signal Processing (ICCSP)*, IEEE, APEC, Chennai, India, pp. 1950–1953.
18. Catarinucci L., Danilo D. D., Luca M., Luca P., Luigi P., Maria L. S., and Luciano T. 2015. An IoT-aware architecture for smart healthcare systems. *IEEE Internet of Things Journal* 2, no. 6, 515–526.
19. Porkodi R., and Bhuvaneswari V. 2014. The internet of things (IOT) applications and communication enabling technology standards: An overview. In *2014 International Conference on Intelligent Computing Applications*, Los Alamitos, CA: Conference Publishing Services, IEEE Computer Society, [2014], pp. 324–329.
20. Kärkkäinen M. 2003. Increasing efficiency in the supply chain for short shelf life goods using RFID tagging. *International Journal of Retail & Distribution Management*, 31(10), 529–536.
21. Na A., and William I. 2016. Developing a human-centric agricultural model in the IoT environment. In *2016 International Conference on Internet of Things and Applications (IOTA)*, IEEE Pune Section and its COMSOC and CS Chapters, Pune, India, pp. 292–297.
22. Zhu C., Victor C. M., Leung L., Shu and Edith C. H. N. 2015. Green internet of things for smart world. *IEEE Access* 3, 2151–2162.
23. Longhi S., Davide M., Emanuele A., Gianluca D. B., Mario P., Massimo G., and Matteo P. 2012. Solid waste management architecture using wireless sensor network technology. In *2012 5th International Conference on New Technologies, Mobility and Security (NTMS)*, IFIP TC6 & IEEE COMSOC, Istanbul, Turkey, pp. 1–5.
24. Welbourne E., Leilani B., Garret C., Kayla G., Kyle R., Samuel R., Magdalena B., and Gaetano B. 2009. Building the internet of things using RFID: The RFID ecosystem experience. *IEEE Internet Computing* 13, no. 3, 48–55.
25. Arshad R., Saman Z., Munam A. S., Abdul W., and Hongnian Y. 2017. Green IoT: An investigation on energy saving practices for 2020 and beyond. *IEEE Access* 5, 15667–15681.
26. Shaikh F. K., Sherali Z., and Ernesto E. 2015. Enabling technologies for green internet of things. *IEEE Systems Journal* 11, no. 2, 983–994.
27. Miorandi D., Sabrina S., Francesco D. P., and Imrich C. 2012. Internet of things: Vision, applications and research challenges. *Ad hoc networks* 10, no. 7, 1497–1516.
28. Fan Z., Georgios K., Costas E., Mahesh S., Mutsumu S., and Joe M. 2010. The new frontier of communications research: Smart grid and smart metering. In *Proceedings of the 1st International Conference on Energy-Efficient Computing and Networking*, New York, United States, Passau Germany, April, 2010, pp. 115–118.
29. Latré B., Bart B., Ingrid M., Chris B., and Piet D. 2011. A survey on wireless body area networks. *Wireless Networks* 17, no. 1, 1–18.
30. Darby S. 2010. Smart metering: What potential for householder engagement? *Building research & information* 38, no. 5, 442–457.
31. Keogh E. 2014. Insect Sensors Target Crop-Eating Bugs For Death. Available: http://www.fastcoexist.com/1679725/insect-sensors-target-crop-eating-bugs-for-death (accessed Jun 19, 2019).
32. McLaughlin M. L., Gaurav S., and Jooao H. 2001. Touch in Virtual Environments: Haptics and the Design of Interactive Systems. Prentice Hall, Imsc Press Multimedia Series PTR, Pearson Education; 1st edition.
33. Idris, M. Y. I., Leng Y. Y., Tamil E. M., Noor N. M., and Razak Z. 2009. Car park system: A review of smart parking system and its technology. *Information Technology Journal* 8, no. 2, 101–113.
34. World Health Organization [Online] http://www.who.int/ (accessed November 07, 2019).

35. International Diabetes Federation (IDF) [Online] http://www.idf.org (accessed November 07, 2019).
36. Ullah S., Pervez K., Niamat U., Shahnaz S., Henry H., and Kyung S. K. 2010. A review of wireless body area networks for medical applications. *arXiv preprint arXiv:1001.0831.*
37. http://fiji.eecs.harvard.edu/CodeBlue (accessed November 07, 2019).
38. http://www.mobihealth.org (accessed November 07, 2019).
39. Al A., Moshaddique N. U., Chowdhury M. S., Riazul Islam S. M., and Kyungsup K. 2012. A power efficient MAC protocol for wireless body area networks. *EURASIP Journal on Wireless Communications and Networking* 2012, no. 1, 33.
40. Ullah S., Henry H., Bart B., Benoit L., Chris B., Ingrid M., Shahnaz S., Ziaur R., and Kyung S. K. 2012. A comprehensive survey of wireless body area networks. *Journal of Medical Systems* 36, no. 3, 1065–1094.
41. Anjum I., Nazia A., Md A. R., Mohammad M. H., and Atif A. 2013. Traffic priority and load adaptive MAC protocol for QoS provisioning in body sensor networks. *International Journal of Distributed Sensor Networks* 9, no. 3, 205192.
42. Javaid N., Sarim H., Mustafa S., Mahmood A. K., Safdar H. B., and Zahoor A. K. 2013. Energy efficient mac protocols in wireless body area sensor networks-a survey. *arXiv preprint arXiv:1303.2072.*
43. Iftikhar M., Nada A. E., and Mehmet S. A. 2014. Performance Analysis of Priority Queuing Model for Low Power Wireless Body Area Networks (WBANs). Procedia Computer Science, 34, pp 518–525. https://doi.org/10.1016/j.procs.2014.07.060, pp. 518–525.
44. Ullah S., Muhammad I., and Mohammed A. 2014. A hybrid and secure priority-guaranteed MAC protocol for wireless body area network. *International Journal of Distributed Sensor Networks* 10, no. 2, 481761.
45. Lee C., Hyung S. L., and Sangsung C., 2010. An enhanced MAC protocol of IEEE 802.15. 4 for wireless body area networks. In *5th International Conference on Computer Sciences and Convergence Information Technology*, November 30 – December 2, in Seoul, Republic of Korea, pp. 916–919.
46. Bradai N., Lamia C. F., Saadi B., and Lotfi K., 2013. New priority MAC protocol for wireless body area networks. In *Proceedings of the 3rd ACM MobiHoc Workshop on Pervasive Wireless Healthcare*, Bangalore, India, Association for Computing Machinery, New York, United States, pp. 1–6.
47. Chakraborty C., Gupta B., and Ghosh S. K. 2013. A review on telemedicine-based WBAN framework for patient monitoring. *Telemedicine and e-Health* 19, no. 8, 619–626.
48. Ahmed A., and Ahmed G. E., 2019. Benefits and challenges of internet of things for telecommunication networks. In *Telecommunication Networks-Trends and Developments*. Rijeka, Croatia: IntechOpen.
49. Aggarwal C. C., and Jiawei H. 2013. A survey of RFID data processing. In *Managing and Mining Sensor Data*,: Editor: Charu C. Aggarwal, Springer, Boston, MA, pp. 349–382.
50. Müllner R., and Andreas R. 2011. An energy efficient pedestrian aware Smart Street Lighting system. *International Journal of Pervasive Computing and Communications, Vol.* 7(2): pp. 147–161.

7

Cyber Security in Terms of IoT System and Blockchain Technologies in E-Healthcare Systems

Sudipta Paul and Subhankar Mishra

CONTENTS

7.1 Introduction

According to Fillit, Rockwood and Young (2016) e-health is "an emerging field in the intersection of medical informatics, public health, and business, which refers to health services and information delivered or enhanced through the Internet and related technologies". From MacIntyre et al. (2018), it is evident that discoveries in genomics, synthetic biology, big data, computer science, etc. have applications in health and medicine. An important matter to be noted is that these converging trajectories are dramatically expanding the repertoire of dual-use technologies which can be harnessed for the benefit of, or harm to, humanity. Some of the threatening situation from using e-health in less secure environments are (Ida, Jemai and Loukil 2016): (a) DOS or gateway attacks, which are malicious attacks on the network preventing communication among the interconnected devices; (b) another risk is overflow of traffic of noisy data in the devices and system network which is enough to shut down the system; (c) another thought-provoking situation where lack of security is threatening is the situation where the hackers benefits from those applications where the security is applicable only to a single device at a time, and for convenience, a weaker encryption system is introduced. Using this situation, the hacker can easily hack into the system to steal the data or to disable the system.

E-Healthcare (Chakraborty, Gupta and Ghosh 2013) involves the use of IoT technologies for better diagnosis and treatment of patients where patients are generally in a remote area or out of reach of direct contact with the doctor. In this context, Remote Patient Monitoring (RPM) at home represents a tempting opportunity for hospitals to reduce clinical costs and to improve the quality of life of both patients and their families. It allows patients to be monitored remotely by means of networks of IoT medical devices equipped with sensors and actuators that collect healthcare data from patients and send them to a cloud-based Hospital Information System (HIS) for processing. Up to now, many different proprietary software systems have been developed as standalone expensive solutions, presenting interoperability, extensibility and scalability issues. An e-health application should be able to provide: (a) whether the situation requires emergency treatment; (b) multimedia conferences; (c) streaming of high-resolution medical images; (d) secure transfer of patient's vital information; (e) confirmation of swift access to e-health data records; and (f) a tele-robotic system.

Nowadays, the Internet of Things (IoT) is a well-known term as the abbreviation for networks of enormous numbers of connected intelligent devices that possess the capability to sense or actuate and are connected to each other via the internet or a local small network. E-healthcare is able to provide the required services because of the underlying network of IoT devices, which are prone to cyber threats. As e-health generates and processes very personal medical data, cyber security is one of the main concerns. Therefore, the main challenge was to determine the process of identifying and filtering the main IoT security theories and privacy concerns which are usable by both the IoT devices and e-healthcare at the same time. After rigorous study, the topics are included here according to their usage in the: (a) end points in the devices; (b) different stages of communication; (c) and also in the application of principles of security of cyberspace in the life-cycle of IoT.

Another technology used in e-health is blockchain, the main underlying technology for bitcoin. It is basically a distributed, shared and decentralized database ledger that stores the transactions and assets over a P2P network. Blockchain can be built as (1) permissioned (or private) network that can be restricted to a certain group of participants, or (2) a permission-less or public network that is open for anyone to join in. Permissioned blockchains provide more privacy and better access control. As it has the potential to provide the distributed and transparent single database with higher security, to every doctor, pharmacist and medical persons simultaneously regardless of the place, time and electronic system, it ensures a better treatment plan from the doctor side, as well as better privacy for the patient's information.

In Figure 7.1, a situation where lack of security in e-health is shown with a precision harm situation. The three main parts of this book chapter are the security of IoT and the blockchain, and their connection with the e-healthcare system. Therefore, it will be a helpful book chapter for future cyber security scientists to identify potential cyber security issues and their mitigation measures. Also, there is an apt discussion about the future elements that should be taken into consideration, given the privacy concerns for IoT in terms of building a unique, robust and universal security system for an e-healthcare system.

Taking account of all the above-mentioned, this chapter is divided into several sections i.e., the IoT Device Life-Cycle, Aspects of Interoperability, Privacy Preservation with Trust

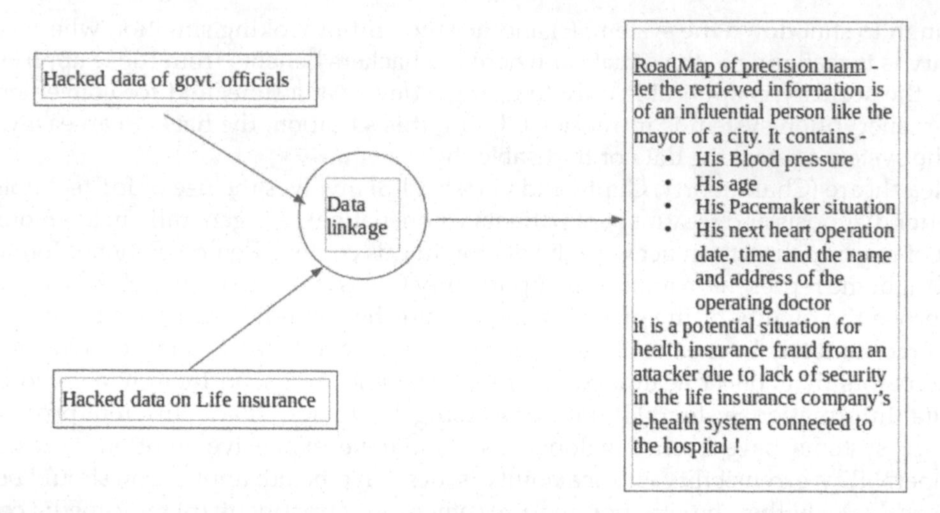

FIGURE 7.1
Situation of precision harm for lack of security in e-health.

and Authentication, Vulnerabilities, Attacks and Countermeasures in IoT, Cryptographical Perspective of IoT security, Cloud Security, Blockchain Technology, Social Awareness, Future Scope and Conclusion.

7.2 The IoT Device Life-Cycle

7.2.1 Introduction

Before discussing the security life-cycle model of IoT devices, we need to know specifically about the functionality of an IoT network (Russell and Van Duren 2016), as well as the workflow among the main functionality. The main functions of IoT take place one by one in the following manner: Sense, Actuate, Profile, Device Management, Control, Application, API, Discovery, Storage, Vertical Analysis, Horizontal Analysis and Translation.

Figure 7.2 shows the functionalities in IoT management. In this chapter, our main concern is specifically around the security part of the IoT Device Management.

The IoT privacy and security challenges are given in Figure 7.3.

As a life-cycle of any working model gives an insight into the workflow of the processes in the system, with its flaws as well as the scope of development, the main components of a security life-cycle of IoT devices (Russell and Van Duren 2016) can be classified as Design, Research and Development, Integration, Operation and Maintenance and Disposal.

Figure 7.4 shows the different stages in the life-cycle of IoT devices. From Figure 7.4, we can easily explain the structure of the security life-cycle in IoT devices as follows.

7.2.2 Explanation of the Different Stages in the Life-Cycle

7.2.2.1 Design

This phase of the life-cycle is specifically intended to propose the structural possibilities with respect to the proper maintenance of the CIA triad (the confidentiality, integrity and

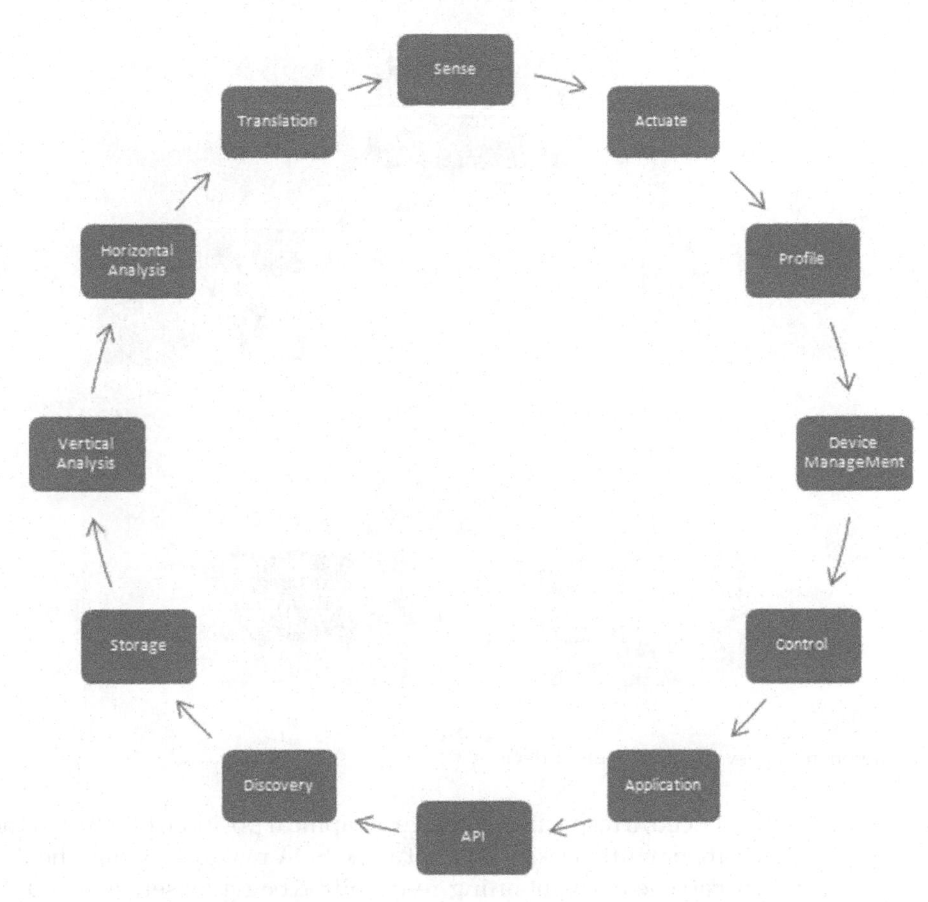

FIGURE 7.2
The Functionalities in an IoT management.

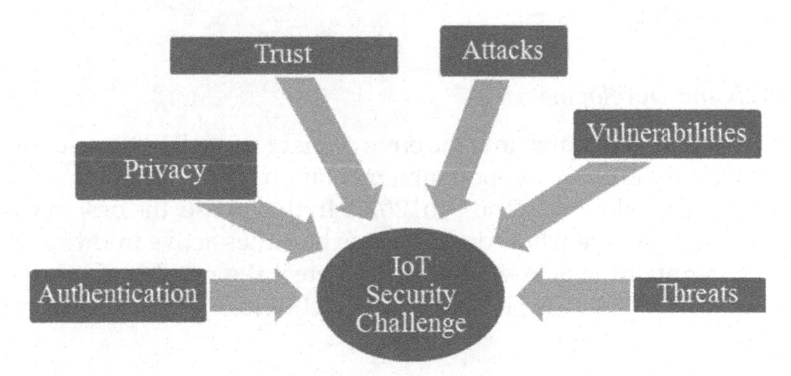

FIGURE 7.3
The security challenges in an IoT device.

availability triad) and Service-Oriented Architecture (SOA). Here, confidentiality means the processes by which it is ensured that the flow of data is not going to an unauthorized person, and also that there is no data manipulation by a person who only has read permission. The main idea of integrity is to maintain the uncorrupted environment throughout the whole life-cycle with respect to data transfer. Here, availability ensures the presence of

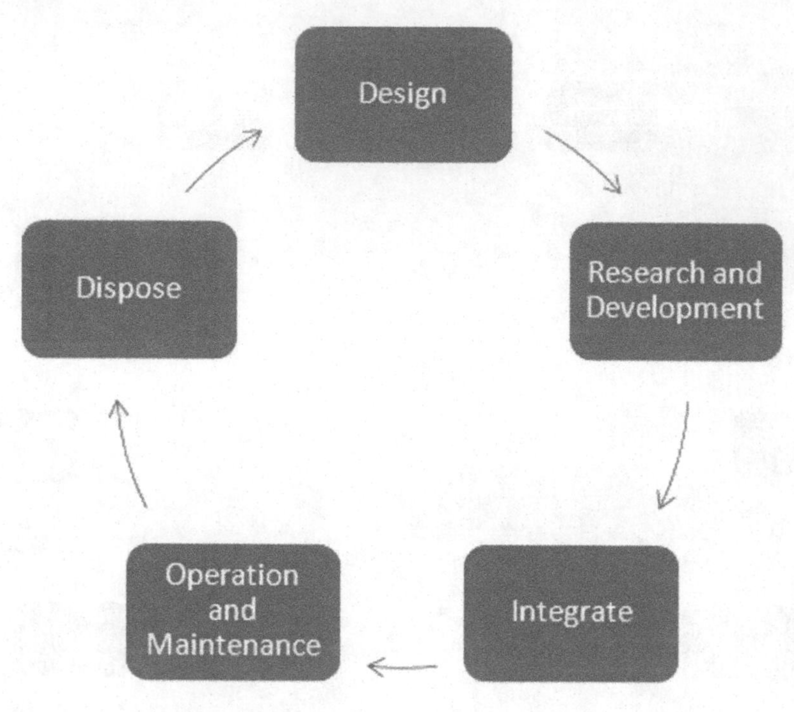

FIGURE 7.4
The main components of device life cycle of IoT devices.

the devices at the time of need, irrespective of the geographical position, glitches in the circumstances, power failure or bottlenecks in the network. SOA makes sure that the devices in the IoT network are capable of maintaining re-usability, being loosely coupled, being location independent and being platform independent, as well as maintaining standards to be an autonomous unit of the IoT network. SOA maintains the device as self-contained, as well as a black box for the users.

7.2.2.2 Research and Development

This phase is dedicated to research into the environment, as well as the user demand at the time of the research, to fulfill the proper implementation of the design phase through programming (Banerjee, Chakraborty and Paul 2019). In this phase, the design would have its physical implementation. The whole design phase becomes active in this phase bit by bit. Also, because of maintaining SOA we can easily detect the problems and disputes in the design phase and correct them as per the current technology and situation in this phase.

7.2.2.3 Integration

In this phase the developed devices connect to each other to make it a proper network. Here the devices then operate and deploy according to their design for further enhancement.

7.2.2.4 Operation and Maintenance

The main function of this stage is managing identities, roles and attributes of the IoT devices as well as monitoring them by naming them with a transparent registration process which is divided into several stages itself on the basis of data-handling sensitivity with respect to compromise impact. The operation phase therefore consists of some interrelated subphases. They can be classified as follows: (a) Identity relationship, management and context; (b) Security monitoring; (c) Penetration testing; (d) Compliance monitoring; (e) Asset and Configuration Management; (f) Incident management; (g) Forensic Management.

The identity relationship, management and context part further works on the basis of attribute-based, role-based and third-party data requirement-based access control to manage the certificates and keys for security. After this phase, security monitoring does its fair share of work to further detect any anomalies or mishaps in the security part. This detection part is further carried out by penetration techniques that take part regularly by following a routine with the help of hardware evaluation and various IoT penetration testing tools like BlueMaho, BlueLog, Crackle, Chibi, Shikra, etc. As the IoT devices are generally made modularly with the mix of different technologies, then each should be taken care of differently with separate updating techniques by maintaining asset and configuration management. The incident management phase is solely responsible for maintaining the critical case histories in the device life and the forensic management part is responsible for the predictive analysis from these data to maintain security in a better way.

7.2.2.5 Disposal

The main concern with the disposal of IoT devices is the possibility of stored data at the time of disposal. In the later section we will see that most IoT devices have a cryptographic layer which can enable the devices to join any network. Also, some devices can store critical data in a range from large to small. Taking account of all these matters, this stage tries to maintain good data archiving and record management with the help of proper inventory control, data warehousing, etc.

7.2.3 Summary

In Sections 7.3, 7.4 and 7.5, we will see that the phases of the life-cycle play the main role in detecting security issues with the framework and architecture of the whole IoT system as well as with a single IoT device in a very significant way.

7.3 Aspects of Interoperability

7.3.1 Introduction

Interoperability means the art or ability of computer systems or smart devices or software to exchange and use the necessary (Peoples 2017) information among or between themselves. Therefore, it is a very important issue in the security cycle of integrating two IoT devices, any two or more intelligent devices or any smart device with the network. The aspects of interoperability therefore can be divided into several aspects:

- **Among Different Internet Protocol Based Layers**

  The main two models in the internet protocol arena (Desai, Sheth and Anantharam 2015) are the OSI model and the TCP-IP model. If we think about the interconnection between these two protocols, then we will see that TCP-IP (IBM's resources for developers and professionals-2018 2018) has four layers from merging some of the layers together from the OSI protocol, which has seven layers. In Figure 7.5 the TCP-IP layers and the corresponding OSI layers are shown: in the essence of IoT networking layers (with respect to TCP-IP layers) there are some definite protocols which will eventually help to establish interoperability (IBM's resource for developers and professionals-2018 2018). They are in Table 7.1. With so many protocols, it is not easy to achieve interoperability. As the sink nodes in the IoT devices are power constrained, they need to have efficient low power networking protocols like Zigbee, Z-Wave, Bluetooth, etc. On the basis of IEEE 802.15.4, Zigbee has been invented; Z-Wave is based on wifi and Bluetooth maintains the IEEE 802.15.1 standard. Three of these protocols are mainly used to establish a small home network using low power radio-wave. There are some differences (Frenzel 2017) between

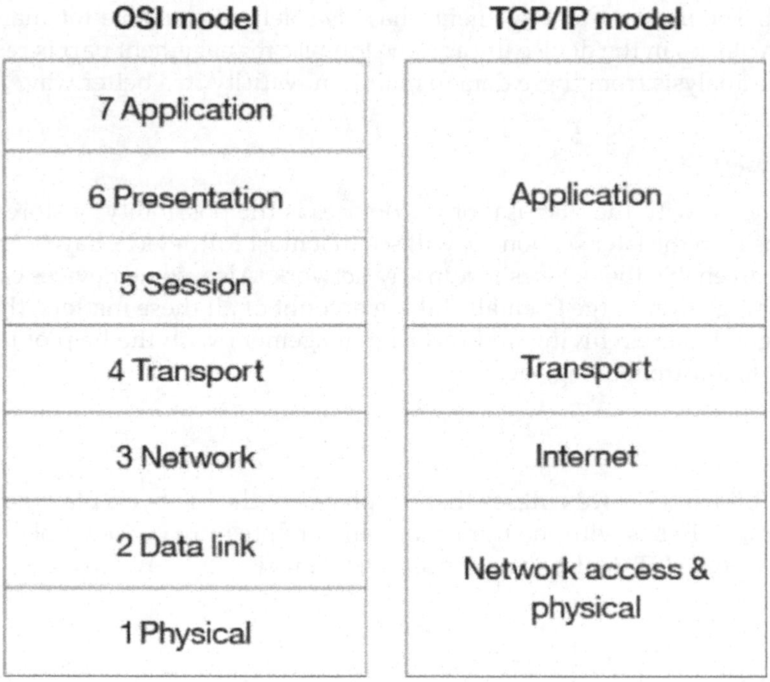

FIGURE 7.5
The OSI layers and their corresponding TCP-IP layers.

TABLE 7.1
IoT Protocols in Different TCP-IP Layers

TCP-IP Model	IoT Protocols
Application Layer	AMQP, CoAP, HTTPS, MQTT, XMPP
Transport Layer	UDP, TCP
Internet Layer	IPv6, 6LoWPAN, RML
Network Access and Physical Layer	IEEE 802.15.4, Wifi (802.11 a/b/g/n), Ethernet (802.3) GSM, CDMA, LTE

Zigbee and Z-Wave too. If we go through the description of these protocols, then we will see that the same general applications are being targeted by ZigBee and Z-Wave. As there will be a great deal of virtually any short-range wireless task in IoT, that's why, of the two, Zigbee is preferable, as it can be configured for these tasks smoothly. For doing the necessary work in a simpler and faster manner, Z-wave is chosen to work with a simpler protocol. The source of Z-Wave chips is Sigma Designs. There are various sources of Zigbee chips like Ember, Freescale, Microchip Technology and Texas Instruments. Complete, ready-to-use Zigbee modules are also available from multiple sources like Atmel, CEL, Digi, Jennic, Lemos and RFM. Z-Wave has a greater range in a given power level when compared to Zigbee, as it uses the Friis formula in the range of 0 dBm power. To produce interference by sharing the ISM band in Bluetooth, wifi and other radio signals, Zigbee generally uses the 2.4 GHz ISM band signal. As Zigbee has co-existence features to help reduce interference, it helps a lot, but it does not compromise the potential of the 908.42 MHz channel of Z-Wave with the help of its 2.4 GHz band.

- **Among Messaging Protocol**
  In Figure 7.5, we can see that the application layer has various de facto standards of messaging protocol i.e., MQTT, CoAP, XMPP, AMQP. An expandable (Desai, Sheth and Anantharam 2015) IoT architecture should be independent of this messaging protocol standard for giving an alliance between various protocols at a time to integrate and translate among themselves for better performance. There are some proposed architectures in the literature that describe the integration between these various messaging protocols seamlessly in a semantic IoT architecture.
- **Among Data Annotation Level**
  There is a lack of interoperability (Desai, Sheth and Anantharam 2015) in this level among the independent devices in various networks. In general, the data are mainly gathered from the sensors, sink nodes, etc. in a raw form. Therefore, it demands extensive manual work to provide a workable form of data with added semantic patterns of metadata. This whole work is done in a bottom-up approach in the IoT network which does not provide any horizontal connection between devices and thus provides the lack of interoperability.

7.3.2 Discussion of Standards regarding Interoperability

7.3.2.1 IPSO (IP Smart Object) Alliance)

The IPSO Alliance (n.d.) is an open, informal association of like-minded organizations and individuals who promote the value of using the IP for networking smart devices with the other devices or with another network. It has announced that they are working on a seamless network to provide communication between every smart object, regardless of its protocol, commissioning, bootstrap, etc. to provide better scalability and interoperability. The messaging protocols used by IPSO are CoAP, LWM2M, IPv6 and MQTT.

7.3.2.2 ETSI (European Telecommunication Standard Institute) Standardization

ETSI (n.d.) is an independent not-for-profit standardization organization in Europe, mainly in the telecommunications industries. It already has 45,784 published standards regarding IoT, especially for telecommunication purposes. The description of the standards is openly available in their website. The different types of standards here mainly depend on the following needs: (a) smoothing trade, (b) enabling economies with efficiency, (c) achieving interoperability and (d) enhancing consumer security

Some of their standardizations are:

- Digital cellular telecommunications system (Phase 2+); Universal Mobile Telecommunications System (UMTS); General Packet Radio Service (GPRS); GPRS Tunnelling Protocol (GTP) across the Gn and Gp interface (3GPP TS 29.060 version 12.6.0 Release 12)
- Universal Mobile Telecommunications System (UMTS); LTE; 3GPP Evolved Packet System (EPS); Evolved General Packet Radio Service (GPRS) Tunnelling Protocol for Control Plane (GTPv2-C); Stage 3 (3GPP TS 29.274 version 12.6.0 Release 12)
- 5 GHz RLAN; Harmonised Standard covering the essential requirements of article 3.2 of Directive 2014/53/EU

7.3.2.3 OIC (Open Interconnect Consortium)

With over 300 member organizations, OIC's aim (*OCF – Open Interconnect Consortium Helps Developers Tackle Internet of Things with New Developer Toolkit* 2017) aim is to provide interoperability standardization to its worldwide member organizations, as well as to all the researchers outside its organization, as a key element to every IoT solution. Some of the big names in the industries such as Samsung Electronics, Microsoft, Electrolux, etc. are members of this organization. Some of its new data models are soundpressure.raml, oic.r, soundpressure.json, GeolocationResURI.swagger.json, etc.

7.3.3 Strength of Interoperability

Here we have mainly discussed IP based system interoperability. The strengths (*Public Safety Tech Topic 2 - Internet Protocol (IP) Based Interoperability* 2015) of it are the following: (a) Resiliency: the internet has a built-in capability of versatility, alternative routing and reliability. This creates a very concrete and backbone interconnection environment for interoperable networks. (b) Scalability: the local network has a limited and simple ability to expand because of a single connection. Therefore, it just becomes a simple addressing issue between the talk groups or the network users. (c) Flexibility: the nature of each network is not a headache to the users because of the only common interface in the network level. Therefore, only one interface is sufficient for different networks. Also, the interconnection is via the internet, therefore all the internet protocols, services, functions and applications can be integrated under one roof across all of the networks. (d) Ease of Development: as the internet protocol network has an open access nature, it allows any number of interconnections at a time. This allows the smooth conversion of the next generation network from previous versions without thinking about issues of interoperability in funding, equipment inventory and versions.

7.3.4 Summary

Interoperability enables IoT devices to communicate more easily. That's why it is done in every layer of an IP configured network to have a better result from every aspect of a device. Also, more and more interoperability is needed in the messaging protocols and in the data annotation level, because exchange of different messaging protocols can enable the mixing up of all types of devices regardless of genre, version incompatibility, storage capacity, etc. This is why the need for universal protocols and frameworks come in the picture. There are many internationally recognized organizations like IPSO, ETSI, OIC, etc. to give such standardizations openly with the help of the industrial organization's or mere users' participation. Thus, we conclude the features of IoT interoperability in a very positive manner.

7.4 Privacy Preservation with Trust and Authentication

7.4.1 Introduction

This whole section is clearly divided into three parts – privacy preservation (Hu 2016), trust and authentication. These three parts are inter-connected. In reality, when a device server tries to connect with another device or another smart system, the whole process should be done privately, revealing only the necessary information from both sides. At the same time the two devices or the two systems should recognize each other on the basis of "trust" to "authenticate" the information that is being received at either side. The following subsections will further discuss these three features (Nzabahimana 2018).

7.4.2 Different Aspects of Privacy Preservation with Discussion of Frameworks

7.4.2.1 Privacy

According to the Oxford English dictionary, the meaning of "privacy" is: (1) freedom from interference or public attention, (2) the state of being alone or undisturbed. Therefore, it is rather a cognitive process and cannot be objectified easily. Thus, boundary and threshold limits of privacy vary from person to person, entirely depending on the effect of the threat. Therefore, the first approach regarding privacy information analysis (Lu et al. 2014) must know its security classification with respect to its privacy attributes (universality and sensitivity). Privacy universality gives the statistical measure from the internet data about "information" that many has thought is to be private, such as the privacy of medical data or bank account data which are considered to be private by everyone. But privacy sensitivity is entirely dependent on the person who owns the information, because the sensitivity is the measure of the amount of secrecy of the data as considered by the data-holder. Therefore the relation between privacy and a privacy breach is the sequence of the following order of arrangement: (a) existence of threat source; (b) the threat source will attack to learn the information; (c) the damage will then be calculated entirely thinking from the user's side with respect to privacy universality and privacy sensitivity. Privacy universality as well as sensitivity are both of two kinds: general and universal universality; general and sensitive sensitivity. If we think of general in both cases as low and universal and sensitive as high, therefore there are four kinds of combination. They are shown in Table 7.2.

Therefore, according to the table there should be three kinds of privacy security level:

Level 1 – both the attributes are general here, therefore the security can be moderate.

Level 2 – either the universality attribute is general or the sensitivity attribute is sensitive, therefore the security is higher than the previous level here.

Level 3 – this level has both the sensitive and universal attributes, therefore it has the highest level of security.

TABLE 7.2
Combination of Privacy Attributes

Privacy Universality	Privacy Sensitivity
General	General
General	Sensitive
Universal	General
Universal	Sensitive

7.4.2.2 Privacy Framework

We will discuss two of the many privacy frameworks here:

1. This architecture is proposed by Bernabe et al. (2014) as a "Privacy-preserving IoT Security Framework". The main components in this framework are: (1) Authentication and Authorization, (2) Identity Management, (3) Group Manager, (4) Key Exchange and Management (KEM), (5) Context Manager and (6) Trust and Reputation. This Bernabe et al. (2014) framework features mainly the Architecture Reference Model (ARM) of IoT-A which is an extension of the traditional ARM security functional group, with more opportunistic and secure sharing models required in an opportunistic IoT that we will discuss in the later section. This framework extends ARM with the help of a context manager to cope with the pervasive and ubiquitous nature of IoT. Here the identity management system ensures privacy management that helps users with means to achieve anonymity, data minimization and unlinkability. The framework introduces a component called Group Manager to deal with more secure and compatible data-sharing models within device users or smart devices or networks.
2. This Kaliya and Hussain 2017) proposed framework addressed the main challenges in privacy preservation in IoT, like a heterogeneous nature, scalability and the need for a common standard for preservation of privacy. Here a framework is to protect users and data with a better classification technique for data with a tag value concept and classification of data on the source value basis. Also, usage of an access control list enabled the framework to ensure data privacy. Users whose access rights are checked are authorized by the server. Therefore, the proposed framework includes data protection and privacy measures with respect to legal frameworks that have relevance to both the protected data and to the final users.

7.4.3 Trust: Its Properties and Objectives with Proper Management

7.4.3.1 Trust Properties

Trust and security are not the same things, but where there is trust there is obviously security. But trust (Yan, Zhang and Vasilakos 2014) is a huge concept with respect to goodness, strength, reliability, availability, ability, or other characteristics of the provider or acceptor of the data. Therefore, trust is a semi-cognitive feature of security. It is hard to maintain, but maintaining it will ensure security properly.

Also, a trustworthy protocol cannot breach the privacy of the users or the provider, ever. Therefore, privacy is also a huge trust property. The main trust properties are therefore the trustee's security and dependability, honesty, benevolence, goodness, being reasonable in relation to the trustor's criteria and policies, the trustor's willingness to work together, the environment and risk of trust, etc.

7.4.3.2 An IoT Trust Management

Trust management consists of: (a) Trust evaluation: this is a technical approach for evaluation of trust for digital processing where the values which can influence trust will be taken into account. Generally, honesty, community interest and co-operative interest are the influencing values here. (b) Trust framework: a trust framework is a kind of system architecture entirely dependent on trust properties to enhance authentication and privacy. (c) Data perception trust: this is the type of trust which comes in handy at the time of data collecting and data preprocessing. The concerns at this stage regarding trust are: whether the data is from the right sensor among multiple sensors, has the sensor not been tampered with, is the sensor verified against relay attack, sensor jamming, replay attack, etc. (d) Identity trust and privacy preservation: this is the part where authentication and integration are being questioned in order to keep it safe. (e) Transmission and communication trust: this type of trust needs to be achieved in order to establish a heterogeneous and specific connection between devices. (f) Secure multiparty computation: this type of trust is all about computation between two parties who are not trusted, but have to be trusted at the time of computation. It is a complete application of computational geometry. It can be achieved in two ways: (1) privacy preserving database query, and (2) privacy preserving data-mining. (g) User trust: this is the study of user behavior which will eventually lead to the success and longevity of the IoT device. (h) IoT application trust: this type of trust comes into the picture when there is a situation where many applications of same type come in the front. One of the approaches is by calculating hash functions to achieve a value and comparing it later.

7.4.4 Authentication

Authentication (Kim and Lee 2017) is a process of identifying an entity which gives away the path to authorization. Authentication is entirely based on trust. If we try to authorize some person based on their ID card, then we have to first trust the issuer, and only after that can we proceed with the authorization part. In the modern IP-networked era (SSL, TLS, PKI, etc.), the CA (certification authority) gives permission to the websites being authorized. Therefore, a cryptographical approach does a huge favor in the time of authentication.

There are several ways of building trust for authentication: (1) Asking a centralized third party trusted authority for a certificate (SSL, TLS, PKI are some of the examples), (2) By using trusted and distributed participants (OPENPGP, LEAP+, Bitcoin, etc. are the examples). Therefore, a locally centralized and globally distributed solution is in demand to process all the challenges in IoT authentication that we can deduce from the above ways of building trust for authentication.

7.4.4.1 Authentication Model Depending on Blockchain

Blockchain (Sedrati, Abdelraheem and Raza 2017) is the main technology implementing the first decentralized cryptocurrency or Bitcoin. It is an optimistic solution to form a feasible decentralized network of IoT with better privacy and security. Satoshi Nakamoto imagined the structure of blockchain. The main agenda of blockchain in security is to provide data integrity, but users' confidentiality or privacy does not concern this technology. As it uses a proof-of-work mechanism (Fabiano 2017), public blockchain-IoT solutions (e.g., IOTA) consume high energy and the number of transactions processed is fewer in comparison to standard payment systems (e.g., VISA). This is why private blockchains with the help of hash-based signatures (e.g., Guardtimes KSI) instead of standard digital signatures provide data integrity fairly. This is the most appropriate choice for IoT applications because the need for a proof-of-work mechanism becomes unnecessary, and this helps to make energy-limited IoT devices to go with symmetric cryptographic operations to join the network.

7.4.5 Summary

From the above discussion we can easily understand the interrelation between privacy, trust, authentication and authorization. They are not a single entity but dependent on each other. Figure 7.6 will give the proper relationship among them.

7.5 Vulnerabilities, Attacks and Countermeasures in the Light of Security Engineering in IoT

7.5.1 Introduction

To understand the vulnerabilities, attacks and countermeasures, at first we need to understand for what purpose they are actually applicable. That is why our first approach will be to understand what information assurance actually is (Russell and Van Duren 2016), as the attacks or vulnerabilities or countermeasures are all circling around this information only. After that we will specifically be going separately into what are actually vulnerabilities, attacks and the measures taken against them in the subsequent subsections.

7.5.2 Information Assurance

To know about information assurance, it is mandatory to know about its components. The components are the following: (a) Confidentiality: the features by which the confidential

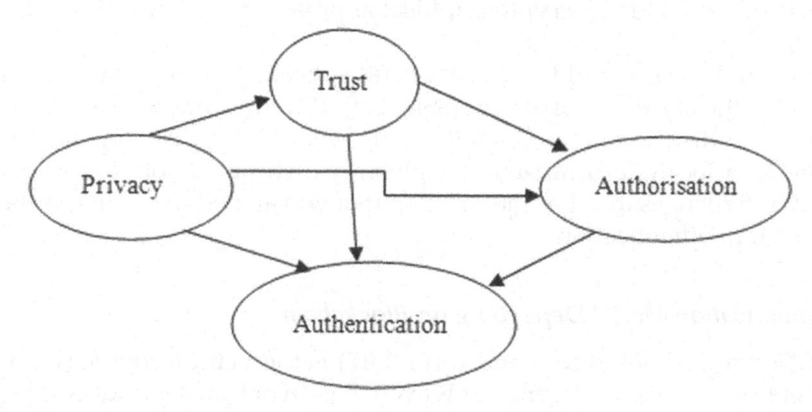

FIGURE 7.6
The interrelation among privacy, trust, authentication and authorization.

information is protected and could not be disclosed; (b) Integrity: unless necessary or detected, the information cannot be changed purposefully according to this feature; (c) Identification and authentication: the source and the destination of the data is verified to be real or fake by this feature. (d) Non-Repudiation: with this feature, a user or a system cannot deny later that the certain action was performed by it. (e) Availability: this feature ensures that the information is always available regardless of its position, network condition, etc.

From the above discussion it is evident that the whole system or the individual devices in an IoT system should go through individual analysis of every piece of data acquired by it because all the data may not possess all the features discussed above. Therefore, an aggregate approach towards information assurance is always desirable, because taking account of a specific measurement towards the set of the same data will always bring good results. In addition to that, another two features are needed to make certain of the information assurance of IoT devices or an IoT system, i.e. (a) Safety: this feature ensures that the system or any of the devices will not go through any harmful situation or not get harmed. (b) Resilience: this feature defines the level of tolerance towards the malicious attacks.

7.5.3 Vulnerabilities

Anything that is a weakness in a system or a device (Russell and Van Duren 2016) can be taken as vulnerabilities. At different stages of the IoT device life-cycle, it will come in different names or shapes like threats or risks, etc. The relationship between each of these concepts is given in Figure 7.7.

From Figure 7.7 the whole process of interdependence of vulnerabilities is treated by proper planning with assessment of the processes and the execution of them. This whole matter of planning can be called "threat modeling" (Qiang et al. 2016). Some features that can be deduced from threat modeling are: (a) in this model, the calculation of effect and cost due to the threats, vulnerabilities, attacks and measurements taken can be calculated; (b) evaluation of target can be measured; (c) the strength of the threat is measured; (d) a priori knowledge of a system or device's vulnerabilities can be measured.

enditemize

7.5.4 Attacks

From the above discussion we can understand that an attack by some intruders is the outcome of these vulnerabilities. Therefore attacks can mainly be differentiated keeping three things in mind (Hu 2016) with respect to the type of vulnerabilities and threats, i.e.

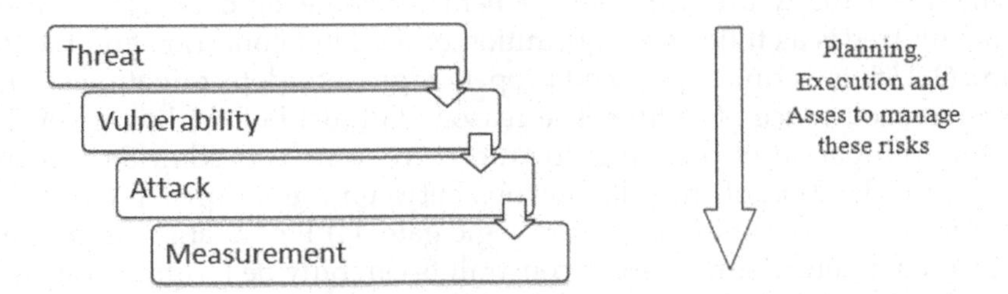

FIGURE 7.7
The interrelation among threats, vulnerability and attack.

(a) Attacks depending on the phases of IoT life-cycle: This attack mainly consist of data leakage or breach, data sovereignty, data loss, data authentication and flooding attack by the intruder. (b) Attacks depending on the Architecture of the IoT network: The main attacks of this kind are external attack, wormhole attack, selective forwarding attack, sinkhole attack, sewage pool attack, witch attack, DDOS (Cusack, Tian and Kyaw 2016) attack, replay attack, sybil attack, byzantine failure, etc. (c) Attacks depending on the components: The main components of an IoT device are terminals, storage and end users, therefore this type of attacks solely target these three main components. At the terminals this attack is mainly in the form of duplication or impersonation of SIM with a virus, worm and revealing of sensitive information. At the storage level, the attack mainly consists of fabrication and disclosure of data. In case of the end users, along with the above-mentioned attack, compromise takes place to mitigate these attacks.

7.5.5 Fault Tree and Attack Tree

After taking account of all types of attack it is time to talk about sorting them in a manageable way (Nagaraju, Fiondella and Wandji 2017) for taking further action in countermeasures. Fault tree and attack tree are two such helpful structures to detect the target of attack or the probability of attack in a step-by-step analysis with the help of a diagram.

7.5.5.1 Attack Tree

Bruce Schneier popularized this term which is basically a tree with a "goal" or attack as the root and the way to "achieve" it as the leaf node (Russell and Van Duren 2016). In this way we can model the threats in a humanly understandable way. In an attack tree, from the bottom up the child nodes are the condition which will eventually satisfy the immediate parent node which may be a child node of another parent node, and finally when the root node is achieved, it is assured that the attack is completed. Therefore, an attack tree is a very good way to trace out the path of a malicious attack to take appropriate measures. Attack tree modeling software are of two kinds, i.e. open source (ADTool of University of Luxemburg, Ent, Seamonster) and commercial (Attacktree+ from Isograph and SecurITree from Amenaza Technologies).

7.5.5.2 Fault Tree

Fault tree (Russell and Van Duren 2016) is a top-down approach to analysis of a failure in a deductive way, using boolean logic for the combination of the lower-level events. It is mainly used to reduce risk or detect a safety accident or a particular failure in a particular level deductively. The fault tree was first introduced in Bell Labs by H.A. Watson in 1962. This tree actually predicts a failure before it can even occur. The process of constructing a fault tree is as follows: (1) Definition of the fault condition and the top level or final failure. (2) Using technical data and proper judgments, determination of the probable reasons for the occurrence of failure. The reasons fall just below the top-level failure in the tree. (3) Continuation of breaking down each reason with additional gates to lower levels. After consideration of the relationships between the failures, the decision will be taken whether to use an "and" or an "or" logic gate. (4) Finalization, and after through revision of the complete diagram, some constraints can only be terminated in a basic fault like human, hardware or software. (5) From this tree structure it is possible to calculate the probability of occurrence of each of the lower-level failures, as well as the bottom-up statistical probabilities.

7.5.5.3 Differences and Collaboration of Fault and Attack Tree

- **Differences**

  The main differences (Russell and Van Duren 2016) between attack tree and fault tree are traversing and entering data in them. If we go through fault tree's features, then by default we will understand the differences between them easily. The features are: (a) Intelligent and well-planned attacks are not the basis of a fault tree formation. (b) They are traversed based on failure rates from each leaf through the dependent intermediate nodes. (c) Each fault tree leaf is completely independent of all other leaves of the tree. (d) Also we can make a fault tree out of an attack tree-making tool by introducing the probability at each level.

- **Collaboration**

  As this collaboration (Russell and Van Duren 2016) concept is still in the literature and experimentation step, we can take a look at some of the recommendations about the collaborations with respect to the above discussion:

  1. In their paper Kumar and Stoelinga (2017) proposed a model which presents attack-fault trees (AFTs), a formalism that combines the security of attack trees with the safety of fault trees. This model is equipped with AFTs having imaginary model checking techniques, which eventually enables an excess of qualitative and quantitative analyses. Qualitative metrics are the main reasons for the system failure, and the quantitative metrics are concerns i.e., likelihood, cost and impact of a disruption. Some of the quantitative measures are: the most likely attack path, the most costly system failure and the expected impact of an attack. To find the attack, the use of sensitivity analysis has the most influence on a metric that gives enough room to justify its workflow.
  2. The protection of Critical Infrastructures (CIs) (Fovino, Masera and De Cian 2009) against security threats and vulnerabilities and the collaboration of fault trees and attack trees against this malicious attack is the basis of this paper. Here they approached the technique of static attack trees, as they did not take account of the time constraint. They also combined a binary decision diagram technique and a Monte Carlo simulation to capture the temporary vulnerable conditions, as there is a lack of databases of complicated attacks regarding temporal conditions, parameters and values of networks.

7.5.6 Countermeasures

From the above discussion we can easily make a "threat model" (Zhang, Cho and Shieh 2015) now for countermeasures to the attacks discussed here. The approximate steps of the threat model are: (a) Identification of the components and assets of the devices in an IoT environment. (b) Construction of the IoT environment architecture. (c) Decomposition of the architecture according to the use. (d) Identification of threats. (e) Documentation of threats using attack and fault trees. (f) Rating the threats by calculating the probabilities from the attack and fault trees.

Using the above model, we can go through component by component to take proper measures using cryptographical steps or cloud security or any other measure which will be proper for the situation as the countermeasure (Russell and Van Duren 2016).

7.6 Cryptographical Perspective of IoT Security

7.6.1 Introduction

Cryptography (Menezes 1997) is the art of studying, practicing and securing the information or data flow in a network in the presence of different attacks, malware, viruses, worms, bugs, etc. to provide an almost lossless network in terms of information. According to R.L. Rivest, cryptography is interesting because of its close tie between practice and theoretical approach with its game-like nature.

This game-like nature assures that the fall of the other side is an inspiration to make the system more developed and secure. Therefore, the main objectives of cryptography can be laid out as follows: (a) Confidentiality or Privacy: The information can be seen only by the authorized person. (b) Integrity of Data: The assurance that information cannot be altered by unauthorized persons. (c) Identification or Authentication with Anonymity: A phase for genuinely identifying an entity (i.e., a person, computer terminal, smartphone, etc.) and concealing it. (d) Data Origin Authentication: Authentication of data source. (e) Signature: A binding method which combines the entity and the information. (f) Timestamp: Taking account of the time of creation of information and the existence of it. (g) Non-repudiation: Prohibiting the denial of previous actions. (h) Certification: Where a trusted third party endorses the authenticity of the information.

7.6.2 Primitives of Cryptography Keeping IoT in Mind

In comparison to computer networks, cryptography does not work through software in IoT devices, but in hardware itself. Also, the main capabilities (Choo, Gritzalis and Park 2018) of an IoT device i.e., data collection, network resource preservation and closed-loop functioning must be preserved through the whole security process. Therefore, the cryptography primitives by which we can assure that the above-mentioned capabilities are intact are discussed in the following.

7.6.2.1 Symmetric Key Cryptography

From Figure 7.8, we can easily understand the process of symmetric key cryptography between two IoT devices. Common symmetric key cryptography ciphers are AES, DES, Triple DES, Blowfish, Camelis, IDEA, etc. From Figure 7.8 it is evident that the main concern in this whole process lies in choosing a key and passing it securely through secured channel. For the "choosing" part, an assumption is made that both the devices know the scheme of their encryption and decryption process beforehand. Therefore, the only data that has to be well-hidden or securely hidden from outsider is the "key"; in Figure 7.8 it is *e*. The decryption key can be easily calculated from the encryption key. Therefore, the load in storage of key in terms of data size is reduced in this process. There are two types of symmetric key cryptography: block ciphers and stream ciphers.

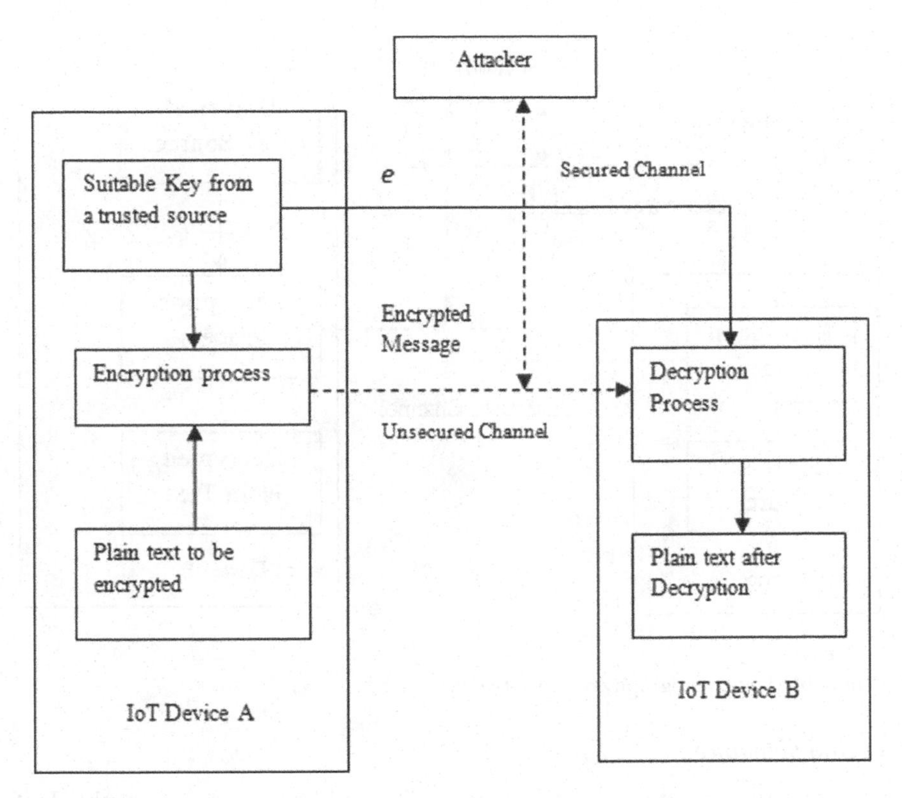

FIGURE 7.8
The process of symmetric key cryptography between two IoT devices.

The main difference between block ciphers and stream ciphers is that stream ciphers are a subset of block ciphers with a block length of one byte, but the reverse is not true. As IoT devices have very limited data buffering, therefore the stream cipher is more efficient for IoT devices. An example of a block cipher is Fiestel Cipher and of a stream cipher, Vernam Cipher.

7.6.2.2 Public Key Encryption

In this type of cryptography there are a set of keys of two types, i.e. a public key and a private key. The whole process of public key cryptography between two IoT devices is depicted in Figure 7.9.

From Figure 7.9 we can easily see that IoT device B selected a pair of two keys i.e., private and public keys. It then sent the public key to the IoT device A over an unsecured channel. Then the encryption process does its job. After that it sends the encrypted message again in an unsecured channel. Then using its private key, IoT device B is able to decrypt the encrypted message uniquely. In the whole process the private key remains secret.

From the above discussion, it is shown that the public key, as well as the encrypted message, travel through an unsecured channel. Therefore, this travel can lead to an impersonation attack if it is not certified to be authenticated and trusted because of the attacker. The solution to this problem lies in the trusted public key technique as well as in the digital signature technique.

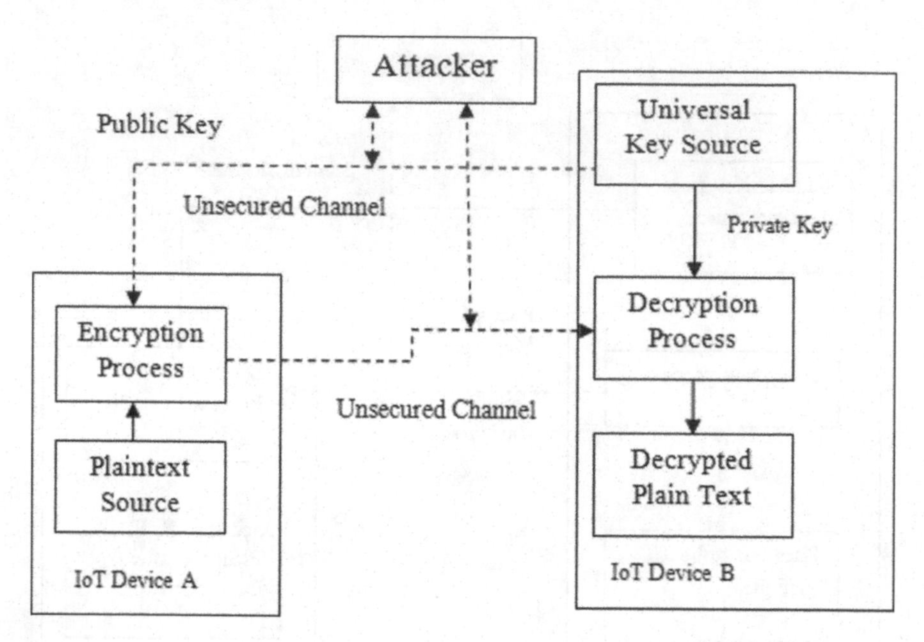

FIGURE 7.9
The process of public key cryptography between two IoT devices.

7.6.2.3 Digital Signature

The digital signature scheme is based on reversible public key cryptography. Just as with a physical handwritten signature, here too the signature is designed to be unique to the signer. Here the signer is the repository of the private signing key and the responsible to sign a message.

After signing the message, the signature will be a part of the message and it will travel to the next step of this scheme. In this step everybody with the right key can do the inverse of the signing or signature verification.

If the signature verification event is successful, then the message will be declared as authentic and not tampered with. But the failure of this event will lead to the message to be declared as tampered with and not authentic, then the message should not be trusted at all. The whole scheme is shown in Figure 7.10.

7.6.2.4 Hashes

A hash function is a very good scheme of cryptography as it maps a variable length of string to a fixed length value called hash value. It is very credible for the following features: (a) It cannot disclose the original message that is being hashed. (b) In this process, two different messages cannot have the same hash values. That defines its uniqueness. (c) The hash values are random-looking. Therefore, the uses of hash function are: (a) Protecting passwords by hashing them into a message digest. (b) Checking the integrity of large dataset by checking the hash values after some time because a hash value for a certain hash function and message string cannot be changed. (c) For performing key generation. (d) To create pseudo-random numbers.

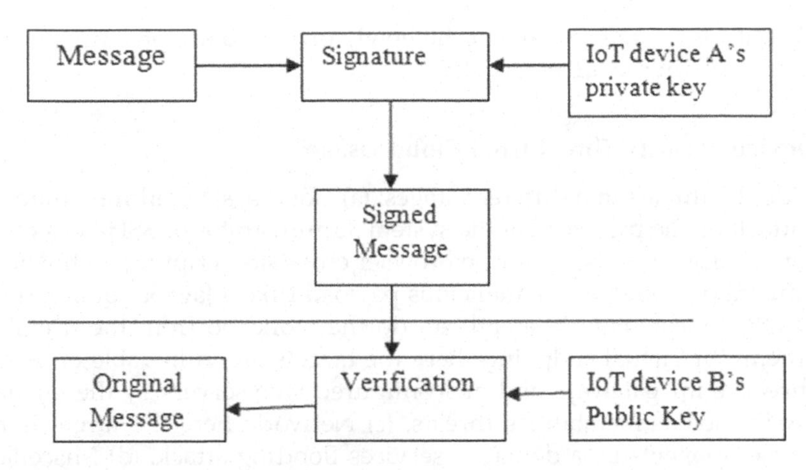

FIGURE 7.10
The process of digital signature between two IoT devices.

7.7 Cloud Security

In order to optimize the full benefits of IoT in the case of e-health, we need the support of the cloud. There are three kinds of clouds to be used in e-health: (1) private, (2) public and (3) hybrid. Here the private cloud is the most secure because only recognized personnel can access the data there. The public cloud is shared and the biggest source of attacks. It is generally shared among different organizations under the control of third-party personnel who are authorized. Hybrid is the combination of both private and public cloud. It uses the best of both worlds and therefore for the part where the data should be stored, it uses the private approach, and the part where the information needs to flow, it uses public part. So both types of security measures are applicable for this kind of cloud architecture. As an example, we can say that the private cloud can be used to store the private information of the patients of that hospital, the public cloud can be used to keep account of the attending doctors of the hospital and the hybrid cloud can be used to store all the private information of the patients who either do not want to disclose it or a patient having AIDS, cancer or something contagious in its private part, and for the public part, it will keep communications among organizations, doctors and patients. In case of cloud security in e-health there are some guidelines and protocols, like HIPAA (Azeez and Van der Vyver 2018) in the US and DISHA in India, etc. ((in draft) Comments on Draft Digital Information Security in Health Care Act. (DISHA): Ministry of Health and Family Welfare: GOI n.d.). Cloud in the case of IoT is mainly used in the back-end of devices for computation purposes. There are other essential uses of the cloud too, like asset or inventory management, service billing and entitlement management, sensor co-ordination, real-time monitoring, data-sharing and message broadcasting, as well as transport and tracking patterns in customer intelligence and marketing (Russell and Van Duren 2016; Hu 2016). Therefore, the cloud has a huge role in security (Koutsouris, Voulkidis and Tsagkaris 2016) of IoT devices. In the subsequent subsections, we will discuss the security threats and controls as well as some of the newly proposed architecture and framework about cloud security in the IoT perspective.

7.7.1 IoT Device Security Threat from Cloud Usage

We can divide the threats into different stages: (a) cloud system administrator and users: dictionary attack on the password of the system administrator or SSH keys to log into the system. There is also a provision of web browser cross-site scripting on the host machine of the administrator. Sometimes a malicious payload (like a JavaScript-based payload) or a malicious attachment sent via email can do the work too from the users' side when they open them. (b) Virtual endpoints: here the targets are vulnerable or misconfigured database, insecure IoT gateways and misconfigured web servers by the virtual machine and web application vulnerabilities threats. (c) Network: here the target is the Virtual Networking Components by a denial of services flooding attack. (d) Miscellaneous: the tampering with and sniffing of traffic, accessing data in the cloud, injecting malicious payloads into the IoT protocols' traffic between devices, edge gateways and cloud gateways of IoT devices, IoT device endpoint spoofing, poor encryption, poor secrecy, insecure database storage on device and theft of IoT devices.

7.7.2 Cloud IoT Security Control

There are many cloud-based industrial IoT security providers like Microsoft Azure IoT suite, AWS IoT, CISCO Fog computing, IBM Watson IoT platform, MQTT and REST interfaces. As the scope of the chapter is small, we are therefore omitting the description of these security providers. But we can take account of the common things or targets of these security providers. (a) Authentication and Authorization: the cloud administrator needs to authorize the authenticity of the individual administrative functions and APIs, end users, cloud applications, IoT devices, its gateways and brokers, proxy authentication of the application users and others. A variety of authentication protocols have been offered by Amazon AWS and Microsoft Azure IoT suite. (b) Software or firmware updating: by updating the software and firmware, the vulnerabilities that occurred in the past can be removed. Therefore, a huge amount of attacks can be prevented by simply updating them. Not only that, but also there should be a mechanism to validate the proper updating of the software and firmware to the end IoT devices. Azure CDN supports automatic software updating. (c) Maintaining data integrity: there are some apt measurements to maintain data integrity, like detecting and preventing the harmful devices from uploading data in the cloud, secured configuration of the gateways at the IoT end by a secure log-in, firewall protection, strong authentication with PKI certificate, etc., updating software. (d) Secure bootstrap and enrolment of IoT devices. (e) Continuous security monitoring with end-to-end security recommendations.

7.7.3 Framework and Architecture

We are going to discuss two architectures that have been proposed in the literature in this section.

1. Memory Efficient Multi Key (MEMK) Generation Scheme:

   The main features of this scheme are: (a) It is a new variant of RSA algorithm. (b) This scheme is especially for the sensitive data from the IoT to cloud and cloud to IoT. (c) With the use of a Diophantine form of non-linear equation this scheme is a proper reuse of the RSA scheme. This is why it does not need to use a multiplicative inverse function or extended Euclidean algorithm. (d) The results are very good from using this scheme by varying the N-bit modulo bits from 1 K to 10 K.

2. In their paper, Stergiou et al. (2018) provide an algorithm by integrating IoT and a cloud security model using an AES and an RSA cryptography algorithm. The result is very good with respect to their speed and rounds.

7.7.3.1 Fog Computing-Based Model

Fog computing (Lee et al. 2015) fills up the hole where the cloud falls short in the IoT environment. The two major structural goals of the fog computing model in IoT technology are (a) Simplification of the development of the network over large decentralized and distributed intelligent devices. (b) The workload of the devices is the key point to dynamically scale the on-demand resources either from fog computing or from the cloud. These two goals improve the quality of services to the user by complementing the shortages that cloud computing provides. As fog computing always provides a latency reserving situation it is a huge research field. In their paper An et al. (2018) have proposed a model using fog computing to protect an IoT system from malicious cyber-attacks. The first step in this proposed system is the adoption of a VPN to ensure secure communications to the IoT devices, and after that it takes an approach to the challenge–response authentication to protect the IoT network strongly from DDoS attacks.

7.7.4 New Scope

The collaboration between cloud and IoT (Russell and Van Duren 2016) has given some new directions for security with its features – software defined networking (SDN), container support for secure development environments, container support for deployment services, microservices and most importantly, the move to 5G connectivity. On-demand computing with dynamic computing resources, cognitive IoT and new trust models for IoT are some of the cloud-enabled directions for IoT which eventually bring a new scope for research.

7.7.5 Summary

From the above discussion, it is evident that cloud computing has been given a new dimension in IoT device security with its own features. Also, it has its own pros and cons with respect to security issues. As this is a huge topic on its own, it therefore has a huge research aspect.

7.8 Blockchain Technology

7.8.1 Introduction

A blockchain is a decentralized, distributed and oftentimes public, digital ledger that is used to record transactions across many computers so that any involved record cannot be altered retroactively without the alteration of all subsequent blocks. This allows the participants to verify and audit transactions independently and relatively inexpensively.

A blockchain database is managed autonomously using a peer-to-peer network and a distributed timestamping server. They are authenticated by mass collaboration powered by collective self-interest. Such a design facilitates a robust workflow where participants' uncertainty regarding data security is marginal. The use of a blockchain removes the characteristic of infinite reproducibility from a digital asset. It confirms that each unit of value was transferred only once, solving the long-standing problem of double-spending. A blockchain has been described as a value-exchange protocol. A blockchain can maintain title rights because, when properly set up to detail the exchange agreement, it provides a record that compels offer and acceptance.

7.8.2 Structure

From the definition of blockchain it is evident that the technology claims to have a transparent and verifiable system in case of exchanging value and sharing data. As it is a distributed ledger it figuratively eliminates the waste of spaces, reduces the fraud risk and creates a transparent system as a whole (Esposito et al. 2018). From Figure 7.11 (Angraal, Krumholz and Schulz 2017) we can easily understand the workflow of a blockchain system. We are skipping the detailed description of a blockchain system architecture; rather, in the following subsection, the main aim is to provide the scenario where this technology is being, or can be, used efficiently while keeping e-healthcare security in mind.

7.8.3 Security Challenges and Probable Remedies

7.8.3.1 Challenges

Healthcare data contains personal and sensitive information that may be attractive to cybercriminals. For example, cybercriminals seeking to benefit financially from the theft of such data may sell the data to a third-party provider, who may perform data analysis to identify individuals who may be uninsurable due to their medical history or a genetic disorder. Such data would be of interest to certain organizations or industries. Therefore, ensuring the security of the EMR/EHR/PHR ecosystem and the underlying systems and components that form the ecosystem is crucial, yet challenging, due to the interplay and complexity between the systems and components. Moreover, the privacy and integrity of healthcare data must be protected not only from external attackers, but also from unauthorized access attempts from inside the network or ecosystem (e.g., employee of the healthcare provider, or cloud service provider). The attacks (e.g., leakage or modification of data) can be intentional or unintentional, and organizations may be penalized or held criminally liable for such incidents, for example, under the US Health Insurance Portability and Accountability Act.

7.8.3.2 A Remedy Model Using Blockchain Technology

Specifically, when new healthcare data for a particular patient is created (e.g., from a consultation, or a medical operation such as surgery), a new block is instantiated and distributed to all peers in the patient network. After a majority of the peers have approved the new block, the system will insert it into the chain. This allows us to achieve a global view of the patient's medical history in an efficient, verifiable and permanent way. If the agreement is not reached, then a fork in the chain is created and the block is defined as an orphan and does not belong to the main chain. Once the block has been inserted into the chain, the data in any given block cannot be modified without modifying all subsequent

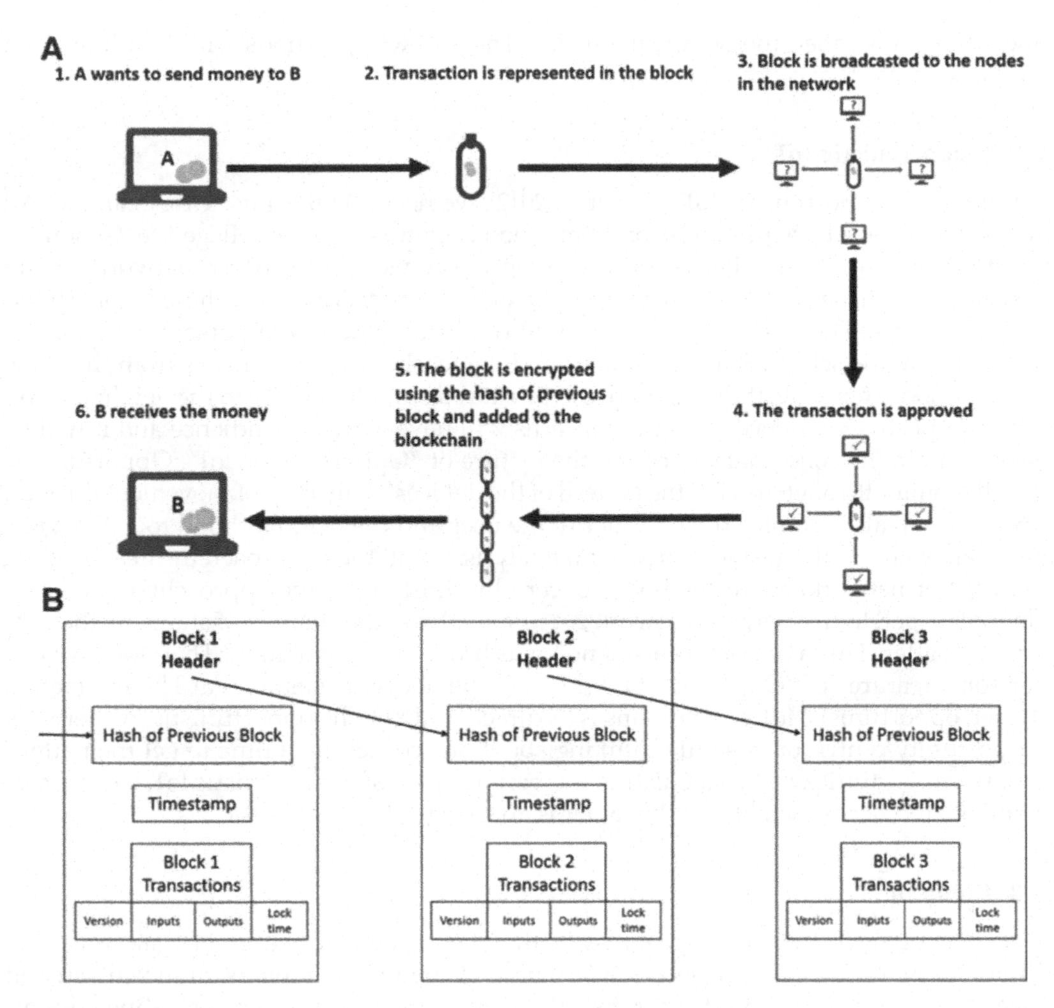

FIGURE 7.11
Workflow of a blockchain system.

blocks. In other words, modification can be easily detected. As block content is publicly accessible, healthcare data needs to be protected prior to the data being in the block (e.g., obfuscated and perhaps encrypted).

7.9 Social Awareness

7.9.1 Introduction

So far, we have only discussed the interaction between the devices or among the networks only. But there is a huge scope of human interaction with the devices or with the IoT network which is explored not that much. This communication between the human and devices is bi-directional, and as IoT is the future of communication, it is more important, based on its social perspectives. As this human interaction with devices has a large opportunity, it is called the opportunistic IoT. The following sections will shed light on it and the concerns that come with it too.

7.9.2 Opportunistic IoT

To understand opportunistic IoT (Guo et al. 2012), we need to take a use case example. All of us at some stage have used a second-hand book in our school or college life. Generally, we get it from our seniors. Let's take a scenario where we have a shared network among the school students and teachers where we can post our concerns about these second-hand book collections. Therefore, the concerns will only stay among the persons who have a relationship to the school. But the students and the teachers are not always from the same neighborhood. Therefore, if the network can be shared simultaneously in the neighborhood of their respective residence, then the concerns will have a greater audience and it will be easier to attain the concern. Here comes the picture of "Opportunistic IoT". Opportunistic IoT will monitor through its GPS the pattern of the devices' daily map of movement through its path. It will also monitor the behavior of the user and the neighborhood too. After getting a pattern from all this monitoring and analysis, it will then approach the nearest node (or device or network) about the book concern by thinking of the approached node as a potential helper. In this way the network got to spread and the chances of attaining the concerns get better. This approach is also known as broker-based solution. Therefore, we can infer some features of "Opportunistic IoT" from the above discussion: (a) The interaction between opportunistic IoT and humans is bi-directional. (b) The opportunistic IoT network is opportunity-centric or it is only thinking about one concern at a time to get the pattern about the opportunity. (c) By calculating the performance of opportunistic IoT, we can easily understand how much human behavior is affecting IoT or vice versa.

7.9.3 Concern

As the network is on the move and it may be that the data provider and the data consumer will not know each other, the security of data and the information assurance discussed above should also be affirmed. Therefore there are some major issues regarding "opportunistic IoT". They are the following: (a) Data distribution protocol: as the data provider node and the consumer node may not be operating in the same time, then a solution can be found by using the capability of the network to store the data by taking the provider and supplying the data at the right time to the consumer in case of any problem on the consumer side. Another option can be making assumptions about the behavior pattern of the human and acting accordingly. For example, taking selfishness as a part of human behavior, we can design attack and failure beforehand and use them as a data distribution protocol at the right time. (b) Establishing relations among divergent social networks: this is a big research area nowadays, as it contains the interaction between the face-to-face communication as well as the interaction between different devices and the human beings and the interaction between different social networking sites from the human sides as well as from different devices. This is a challenging research area because of the difficult features of human behavior patterns regarding social sites. These social sites also have different features with respect to network support, geographical location, sound, cloud security, etc. Therefore, mixing together all these constraints and not to overdoing something is a great research challenge itself. (c) Security: the main concern here is to preserve the privacy of the data, device and the participants in the opportunistic IoT network, as well as giving an opportunity to the devices and the participants to have a smooth flow of information without any breach of security and trust. One of the measures regarding this matter is using an anonymous data provider who is authenticated by some online authentication servers. This is not credible all the time because of the threat and trust model analysis we have discussed before. This is why it is a huge subject of research. (d) Necessity of generic structure: as the scope of the opportunistic IoT is huge but the functional capabilities of the devices and human beings are limited, there should therefore be a generic structure, by using which the working function can be of proper use. The structure should provide a dynamic environment for essential protocols to share the mobile nodes effectively without jeopardizing the above-mentioned concerns. It is also a huge research topic nowadays. Guo (2012) has proposed such an architecture.

7.10 Future Scope and Conclusion

In the above discussion we have seen in case of e-health how the IoT devices work together with other devices in a network during its lifetime. Also, it is shown how the phenomenon of interoperability may eventually lead an IoT device to some serious privacy and security attacks, as interoperability ensures free mixing up of devices by (sometimes) compromising its peripheral situation. As the problem arises, the question of solutions is also raised. To come to a solution, one needs to know the characteristics of the attack and the threat and vulnerabilities regarding the situation. After learning about the situation fully, then it is time to proceed with the countermeasures. Here we have mainly studied the cryptographical, cloud and social perspective of IoT devices' security and privacy problem solutions in the light of e-health. Therefore all of these are mainly software solutions. To get a thoroughly secure IoT environment, the need for securing objects and devices from software as well as hardware is very much essential.

The regrettable matter is that researchers have been relentlessly identifying the security flaws one by one till now in IoT networks and devices, but due to a lack of proper databases and experience in solving these kinds of problems, there were no concrete standard solutions that could overcome all those problems at once till now. IoT security is the area concerned with secure embedded devices connected to IoT systems. This area is important to prevent important data loss or corruption. A good security level for IoT devices is the way to achieve new business opportunities too. In the case of blockchain (Esposito et al. 2018), the main problem is the data integrity and the large size of data. As the original technology is merely for swift transactions and healthcare data has a huge size, the fit of the technology needs more research in the future. A probable solution for the latter matter is to use off-chain storage. Further research can be done in that direction.

Therefore, for future work we need to think of a way where a concrete solution regarding hardware and software will give a unanimously standard suit as software threats and hardware threats are dependent on each other. So, to have a robust e-health framework there should be a proper collaboration globally among health personnel, law enforcement, defense and intelligence agencies with cyber specialists having a common ground with new risk analysis methods and strong surveillance methods. The main agenda of that solution will entirely be dependent on the following elements: (a) information assurance, (b) universal interoperability, (c) highest interdependency of software with hardware and vice versa, (d) universal authentication process, (e) no compromise in the trust section, and (f) having more social awareness, etc.

References

(N.d.). https://en.wikipedia.org/wiki/IPSO_Alliance.

(N.d.). https://www.etsi.org/about.

An, Xingshuo et al. (2018). Hypergraph clustering model-based association analysis of DDOS attacks in fog computing intrusion detection system. *EURASIP Journal on Wireless Communications and Networking* 2018(1), 249.

Angraal, Suveen, Harlan M. Krumholz, and Wade L. Schulz (2017). "Blockchain technology: applications in health care". *Circulation. Cardiovascular Quality and Outcomes* 10(9), e003800.

Azeez, NureniAyofe and Charles Van der Vyver (2018). "Security and privacy issues in e-health cloud-based system: A comprehensive content analysis". *Egyptian Informatics Journal* 20(2), 97–108.

Banerjee, Sourav, Chinmay Chakraborty, and Sudipta Paul (2019). "Programming Paradigm and Internet of Things". In *A Handbook of Internet of Things & Big Data*, pp. 148–164, CRC Press, Taylor and Francis

Bernabe, Jorge Bernal et al. (2014). "Privacy-preserving security framework for a social-aware internet of things". In *International Conference on Ubiquitous Computing and Ambient Intelligence. Springer, pp.* 408–415.

Chakraborty, Chinmay, B. Gupta, and S. K. Ghosh (2013). "A Review on Telemedicine-Based WBAN Framework for Patient Monitoring, Int. Journal of Telemedicine and e-Health". *International Journal of Telemedicine and e-Health* 19(8), 619–626.

Comments on Draft Digital Information Security in Health Care Act. (DISHA): Ministry of Health and Family Welfare: GOI (n.d.).

Cusack, Brian, Zhuang Tian, and Ar Kar Kyaw (2016). "Identifying DOS and DDOS attack origin: IP traceback methods comparison and evaluation for IoT". In *Interoperability, Safety and Security in IoT*. Springer, pp. 127–138.

Desai, Pratikkumar, Amit Sheth, and Pramod Anantharam (2015). "Semantic gateway as a service architecture for IoT interoperability". In: *Mobile Services (MS), 2015 IEEE International Conference on*. IEEE, pp. 313–319.

Esposito, Christian et al. (2018). "Blockchain: A panacea for healthcare cloud-based data security and privacy?" *IEEE Cloud Computing* 5(1), 31–37.

Fabiano, Nicola (2017). "The Internet of Things ecosystem: The blockchain and privacy issues. The challenge for a global privacy standard". In *Internet of Things for the Global Community (IoTGC), 2017 International Conference on*. IEEE, pp. 1–7.

Fillit, Howard M., Kenneth Rockwood, and John B. Young (2016). *Brocklehurst's Textbook of Geriatric Medicine and Gerontology E-Book*. Elsevier Health Sciences.

Fovino, Igor Nai, Marcelo Masera, and Alessio De Cian (2009). "Integrating cyber attacks within fault trees". *Reliability Engineering & System Safety* 94(9), 1394–1402.

Frenzel, Lou (2017). *What's the Difference Between ZigBee and Z-Wave?* https://www.electronicdesign.com/communications/what-s-difference-between-zigbee-and-z-wave

Guo, Bin et al. (2012). "Opportunistic IoT: Exploring the social side of the internet of things". In *Computer Supported Cooperative Work in Design (CSCWD), 2012 IEEE 16th International Conference on*. IEEE, pp. 925–929.

Hu, Fei (2016). *Security and privacy in Internet of things (IoTs): Models, Algorithms, and Implementations*. CRC Press.

IBM's resource for developers and IT professionals-2018 (2018). *IBM developer Works, Learn, Develop, Connect* www.ibm.com/developerworks/index.html

Ida, Imen Ben, Abderrazak Jemai, and Adlen Loukil (2016). "A survey on security of IoT in the context of eHealth and clouds". In *2016 11th International Design & Test Symposium (IDT)*. IEEE, pp. 25–30.

Kaliya, Neha and Muzzammil Hussain (2017). "Framework for privacy preservation in IoT through classification and access control mechanisms". In *Convergence in Technology (I2CT), 2017 2nd International Conference for*. IEEE, pp. 430–434.

Kim, Hokeun and Edward A. Lee (2017). "Authentication and Authorization for the Internet of Things". *IT Professional* 19(5), pp. 27–33.

Koutsouris, Nikos, Apostolos Voulkidis, and Kostas Tsagkaris (2016). "A framework to support interoperability in IoT and facilitate the development and deployment of highly distributed cloud applications". In: *Interoperability, Safety and Security in IoT*. Springer, pp. 41–48.

Kumar, Rajesh and Marielle Stoelinga (2017). "Quantitative security and safety analysis with attack-fault trees". In *High Assurance Systems Engineering (HASE), 2017 IEEE 18th International Symposium on*. IEEE, pp. 25–32.

Lee, Kanghyo et al. (2015). "On security and privacy issues of fog computing supported Internet of Things environment". In: *Network of the Future (NOF), 2015 6th International Conference on the*. IEEE, pp. 1–3.

Lu, Xiaofeng et al. (2014). "Privacy information security classification study in internet of things". In: *Identification, Information and Knowledge in the Internet of Things (IIKI), 2014 International Conference on*. IEEE, pp. 162–165.

MacIntyre, C Raina et al. (2018). "Converging and emerging threats to health security". *Environment Systems and Decisions* 38(2), 198–207.

Menezes, Alfred J (1997). *Handbook of Applied Cryptography/Alfred J. Menezes, Paul C. van Oorschot, Scott A. Vanstone.*

Nagaraju, Vidhyashree, Lance Fiondella, and Thierry Wandji (2017). "A survey of fault and attack tree modeling and analysis for cyber risk management". In *Technologies for Homeland Security (HST), 2017 IEEE International Symposium on*. IEEE, pp. 1–6.

Nzabahimana, Jean Pierre (2018). "Analysis of security and privacy challenges in Internet of Things". In *2018 IEEE 9th International Conference on Dependable Systems, Services and Technologies (DESSERT)*. IEEE, pp. 175–178.

OCF – Open Interconnect Consortium Helps Developers Tackle Internet of Things with New Developer Toolkit (2017). https://openconnectivity.org/news/open-interconnect-consortiumhelps-\newlinedevelopers-tackle-internet-of-things-with-new-\newlinedevelopertoolkit-2.

Peoples, Cathryn (2017). "A Standardizable Network Architecture Supporting Interoperability in the Smart City Internet of Things". In *Interoperability, Safety and Security in IoT*. Springer, pp. 38–45.

Public Safety Tech Topic 2 - Internet Protocol (IP) Based Interoperability (2015). https://www. fcc.gov/help/public-safety-tech-topic-2-internet\newline-protocol-ip-basedinteroperability.

Qiang, Li et al. (2016). "Framework of Cyber Attack Attribution Based on Threat Intelligence". In *Interoperability, Safety and Security in IoT*. Springer, pp. 92–103.

Russell, Brian and Drew Van Duren (2016). *Practical Internet of Things Security*. Packt Publishing Ltd.

Sedrati, Anass, Mohamed Ahmed Abdelraheem, and Shahid Raza (2017). "Blockchain and IoT: Mind the Gap". In *Interoperability, Safety and Security in IoT*. Springer, pp. 113–122.

Stergiou, Christos et al. (2018). "Secure integration of IoT and cloud computing". In *Future Generation Computer Systems* 78, pp. 964–975.

Yan, Zheng, Peng Zhang, and Athanasios V. Vasilakos (2014). "A survey on trust management for Internet of Things". *Journal of Network and Computer Applications* 42, 120–134.

Zhang, Zhi-Kai, Michael Cheng Yi Cho, and Shiuhpyng Shieh (2015). "Emerging security threats and countermeasures in IoT". In *Proceedings of the 10th ACM Symposium on Information, Computer and Communications Security*. AC Med, pp. 1–6.

8

Domestic Medical Tourism for National Healthcare Systems

Sukanya Roy

CONTENTS

8.1 Introduction

In the present era, the definition of "health" is explained by the WHO (World Health Organization) "as a state of complete, physical, mental and social well-being, not merely the absence of disease or infirmity". Health is a complete state of emotional and physical well-being. The importance of the healthcare system is to provide quality healthcare services to all people without any unfairness. In the current context, the concept of "medical tourism", where patients travel globally to obtain the best medical care at a low cost, is highly in demand. In India, medical tourism is the fastest-growing sector, according to the reports of the Ministry of Health, stated that in 2017, 495,056 patients visited India to seek medical care. The reason behind the phenomenon of growing medical tourism in India is largely the infrastructural development, multi-specialty hospitals and investments that were made to boost medical tourism in India. Apart from these, a study conducted by Singh and Badaya (2014) proposed that in the healthcare system there is a huge gap between "need and feed" that can be seen in rural India. Lack of quality in healthcare services and poor medical infrastructure leads these rural people to travel from their hometowns toward the cities to get primary medical treatment. Domestic medical tourism is a modern concept where patients travel to cities to get the best medical treatment from city hospitals. The present chapter broadly discusses the neglected aspect of domestic medical tourism in rural India. Several past studies found that global health tourism has a huge impact on the economic benefits which are created by the overseas tourist (Bookman and Bookman, 2007). Similarly, studies mainly contribute in the areas on international medical tourism, whereas few studies have captured data on the area of domestic medical tourism, which is usually found in rural India as compared to urban areas. The main reason behind medical tourism in rural India is due to unsuitable medical facilities and poor health infrastructure. The present study mainly identifies: (a) the pain points of the domestic tourists, especially the patients from rural India who hope to access better medical facilities in city medical hospitals, and (b) it identifies the "medical tourist's" expectations choosing urban hospitals as medical tourism destinations.

8.2 Medical Tourism

Medical tourism is also known as medical travel, health tourism or global healthcare. In the present era medical tourism is in high demand, with patients traveling globally to access better healthcare facilities (Eissler and Casken, 2013). According to Carrera, medical tourism is defined as organized travel outside someone's healthcare jurisdiction to enhance or restore health. The rise of medical tourism largely depends on two factors: (a) individual-related factors, and (b) provider-related factors which were subcategorized into many elements like doctor's availability, budget, certification and accreditation, accessibility and communication (Oberoi and Kansra, 2019). According to the Hastings Center Report (2010), Cohen suggested three types of medical tourism:

a) Medical tourism for services that are illegal in both the patient's home country and the destination countries.
b) Medical tourism for services that are illegal in the patient's home country, but legal in the destination countries.
c) Medical tourism for services that are legal in both the patient's home country and the destination countries.

Table 8.1 describes a literature survey of medical tourism by the authors.

8.3 Important Factors behind the Growth of Medical Tourism

Medical tourism broadly defined as travel that mainly focuses on medical treatments. Bookman and Bookman (2007) have defined medical tourism as a journey to improve health, and it includes two sectors: medicine and tourism. The major contributing factors which impact the growth of medical tourism in emerging nations, especially in India, are standard medical services with lower costs. Han et al. (2018) postulated that medical tourism largely covers health services like dental, cosmetics and other specialist treatments. Oberoi and Kansra (2019) believe that medical tourism is mainly influenced by two factors: individual-related factors and provider-related factors. The individual-related factors were broadly classified into country selection, hospital selection and doctor availability,

TABLE 8.1

Definitions of Medical Tourism

Authors	Definitions
Goodrich and Goodrich	Defined healthcare tourism as "the attempt on the part of a tourist facility or destination to attract tourists by deliberately promoting its healthcare services and facilities, in addition to its regular tourist amenities" (p.217)
Gupta	According to Gupta, "well-defined medical tourism is the endowment of the cheap medical facility for patients in alliance with the tourism industry"
Carrera	Medical tourism is defined as an organized journey outside of someone's healthcare jurisdiction to enhance health (p.1453)
Whittaker	According to Whittaker, medical tourism is considered as a synonym for health tourism
Gupta and Das	According to Gupta and Das, medical tourism is an activity where individuals travel to other countries for healthcare services such as dental, surgical and medical which are either not available or are highly expensive in patients' countries
Glinos and Baeten	According to Glinos and Baeten, medical tourism is the activity of a patient who moves overseas to seek healthcare services because of some relative disadvantage in their own nation's healthcare system

whereas provider-related factors were sub-categorized into infrastructure, certification and accreditation and accessibility and communication. According to Grail (2009) and Yu et al. (2011) the prime six factors which increase the attractiveness of medical tourism are (a) affordability, (b) alternative and innovative therapy, (c) better quality care, (d) aging population, (e) long waiting times and (f) a large uninsured population. A similar study by FICCI (2016) recognized the major drivers for medical tourism in India as medical "(quality, reliability & credibility and adequate infrastructure), economical (insurance coverage, low cost) and social & technology (internet, privacy, and culture, etc.)". From a previous study, it was stated that the growth of medical tourism is driven by many factors. Musa et al. (2012), examined the motivation behind the traveling tourist. By conducting a research study, the authors inferred that the key determinants were money, excellent medical services, support services and cultural similarity. These were the prime motivational factors behind the medical tourist. Tourists primarily select the country location and other demographic factors and then look for a medical facility, infrastructure and service availability (Kim). In addition, study conducted by Caballero-Danell and Mugombo (2007) postulated that customer benefits, branding communication channels, legal framework and infrastructure are key drivers which draw the attention of healthcare tourists. A similar study by Ye et al. (2008) recognized elements like "marketing promotion programs, cost, communication, employee expertise and certification" which encourage the medical tourist to visit the destination for healthcare services. Exploring previous studies, it investigated the factors which motivates the patient to seek an international destination for treatment. Hence, from the past literature review, it has been easier to recognized and categorize factors such as "doctor availability, infrastructure, accreditation and certification, and communication" as the prime determinants to influence medical tourism (Oberoi and Kansra, 2019).

8.4 Medical Tourism: Emerging Trends

Past studies (Hudson and Li, 2012; Connell, 2006) showed that the growing popularity of medical tourism is largely found in emerging markets like Thailand, Malaysia and India.

There are certain attributes which influence the patient's decision to access healthcare facilities in these emerging countries. Modern healthcare facilities, skilled doctors and low-cost treatments have made India the most popular hub for domestic medical tourism. In the present scenario, India recently became the prime destination for medical tourists. As stated by Hyder et al. (2019) medical tourism in emerging countries is entirely based on trust, positive word of mouth and a network build by the healthcare providers. The rise of medical tourism in emerging countries leads to economic growth (Bookman and Bookman, 2007).

8.5 Healthcare Market Size

The healthcare industry in India includes "hospitals, medical devices, clinical trials, outsourcing, telemedicine, medical tourism, health insurance, and medical equipment" (Akriti Bajaj, Invest India: Chakraborty et al., 2013). According to the IBEF report, the market size of the healthcare industry in 2018 was $150 billion which was expected to grow by "USD 372 billion by 2022" and the key factors behind the rapid growth in the healthcare market are lifestyle diseases and the rising demand for affordable healthcare delivery systems. In the present era, the nation is witnessing a new type of increase in Indian hospitals, due to what is known as medical tourism. Medical tourism is the most important part of the healthcare sector. As per a report titled "India: Building Best Practices in Healthcare Services Globally, 2019" published by the Federation of Indian Chambers of Commerce and Industry (FICCI) and Ernst & Young stated that the medical tourism market is expected to touch $9 billion by 2020.

8.6 Medical Tourism Industry Perspective

Medical tourism is an important part of the healthcare sector in India, which has a unique combination of advanced facilities and skilled doctors with low treatment costs which have led to the nation being considered the most popular hub of medical tourism. Health tourism is a multi-billion-dollar industry that is promoted by the Indian government and nourished by the corporate boom in medical care. This is because the rise in medical tourism has a huge impact on national economic activities that involve the services industry (Bookman and Bookman, 2007).

A report titled "India: Building Best Practices in Healthcare Services Globally 2019" published by Ernst & Young and the Federation of Indian Chambers of Commerce and Industry (FICCI) showed that India is growing as the most preferred destination of "medical tourists". Medical tourism is largely divided into two domains: global tourism and domestic tourism. A study conducted by Baksi and Verma indicated 7.5% of domestic medical trips were to other states and 15% of domestic medical trips were outside states to urban areas. From the above statistics, we can conclude that India is a huge market for both global and domestic medial tourists.

8.7 Domestic Medical Tourism

It was Hudson who first introduced the concept of domestic medical tourism. Domestic medical tourism is the practice of traveling from one city to another or from one state to another within one's country for medical treatment. Glatter proposed that in the future, "domestic medical tourism [will be] a new paradigm of how the best medical care can be stained at the lowest cost. Most primarily the concept of domestic medical tourism, the focus will be on the quality of healthcare delivery rather than on low cost". Several past studies captured factors that the rise in demand for domestic tourism by rural residents in India which were described in the following points. A study conducted by Baksi and Verma proposed that the lack of poor health infrastructure is the major reason for moving to access better medical treatment from urban hospitals. Apart from poor medical infrastructure, there is a unique trio of factors in combination – high-quality medical facilities, proficient regional-speaking medical professionals and low medical costs – which are a vital reason for the rise of domestic medical tourism. In the present chapter, the author discussed the patients' expectations in the context of domestic medical tourism. An expectation is a strong belief that considers something will happen in the future. Expectation concerning the healthcare system is a strong belief that patients will encounter in a healthcare system. Patients will consult a doctor with lots of expectations. The study conducted by Lateef (2011) explains the term patient expectation: "Expectations, regarding health care, refer to the particular belief about what is to be encountered in a consultation or the healthcare system, it is the mental picture where patients will have in the process of interaction with the system". According to the study by Moral et al. (2007) showed that patients with unmet expectations will never follow up care with the consultant; this leads to the conclusion that the trust has been lost in the patients' eyes. Past studies (Kravitz et al., 1994; Ruiz Moral et al., 2007) found that the most common expectations were that the healthcare provider will understand and talk about problems and doubts with the patients. Truner et al. (1998) considered information on pain management and discussing how to return to normal life. Several past studies discussed the number of patients' expectations. Similarly, patients have expectations for domestic medical tourism. Expectations about healthcare relate to beliefs about the healthcare system and about doctors (Lateef, 2011). It a mental picture that is held by the patients during the process of interaction. Lateef (2011) explained patient expectations were categorized into two elements: a) value-based care, and b) patient-centered care. Javed examined the impact of the five service qualities (empathy, responsiveness, tangibility, reliability and assurance) on Pakistani expectations, and the study found that patient satisfaction is strongly associated with empathy in the public sector and responsiveness in the private sector. Adugnaw et al. proposed that post-consultation expectations have a major influence on patient satisfaction. Several studies on the global health tourism captured economic benefits as well as the expectations of the global patients, but few studies highlight the expectations of the domestic medical tourists. The expectations of domestic medical tourists have been discussed in this chapter.

8.8 Methodology

The present study design was a qualitative investigation that involves face-to-face and telephone interviews with the patients who frequently visit Jaipur for treatment. The research methodology was again subdivided into three sections:

a) **Participant Recruitment**

Patients were enrolled through multi-specialty hospitals in Jaipur, as a large proportion of registered patients had already self-identified as "rural domestic patients". Purposive sampling was carried out for the present research. Cresswell notes that purposive sampling seeks participants and help to understand the research problems. According to this, participants were included if they were over 18 years of age and self-identified as "rural domestic patients".

In total, 14 patients were enrolled between August and the first week of October 2019. Enrolment occurred alongside data collection and ended when researchers found that data saturation had been achieved.

b) **Data Collection**

Interviews were carried out by the researchers at Jaipur multi-specialty hospitals. Interviews were recorded for transcription later. The audio-recordings of the interviews were transcribed verbatim and then checked thrice to ensure accuracy by the researchers, but were not returned to respondents for checking. Each interview lasted for 30–40 minutes.

Selection Factors: All services have a series of qualitative specifications which have different combinations of the attributes that represent a different variety of services.

a) **Independent Variables:** Price, availability of specialist doctor, accommodation and healthcare quality (Yu et al., 2018).
b) **Research Context:** The study was mainly conducted in the capital city of Jaipur, Rajasthan where large numbers of rural tourists from the adjacent villages, and Tier 2 and Tier 3 cities visit for health check-ups.

The main hospitals of Jaipur city which drew attention from the domestic tourists:

a) SMS Hospital
b) Fortis
c) Manipal Hospital
d) Dunlopji
e) Tongiya Hospital
f) Mahatma Gandhi Hospital
g) Bhagwan Mahaveer Cancer Hospital

c) **Selection Factors:** The selection of the respondents was made on socio-demographic factors like age, occupation and gender.

8.8.1 Results

Data Analysis: The study included an in-depth interview of all 14 respondents.

Table 8.2 provides a detailed explanation of the socio-demographic of participants.

Demographic analysis of the results concluded that the gender breakdown was 57% female and 43% males and from the data it is revealed that the most popular services for Indian medical tourism are cardiac, gynecology and orthopedics. Apart from this, oncology is the next most popular specialty which is accessed by the patients. From the qualitative data, it has been found that Jaipur is the most preferred domestic medical tourism destination for the nearby Tier 2 and Tier 3 cities. The data has revealed that more than 50% of patients have to fund their medical treatment themselves, followed by those who were government-sponsored (Bhamashah Card) and those who had private health insurance.

Data Analysis

The thematic framework method of analysis was applied. The whole analysis occurred in six steps:

TABLE 8.2

Socio-Demographic Description of Respondents

Gender	Age	Occupation	Financial Support	Medical Tourism Product
M	7	NA	Self-financed	Pediatrician
F	25	Homemaker	Self-financed	Gynecologist
M	60	Family business	Government-sponsored (Bhamashah Card)	Cardiologist
M	6	NA	Self-financed	Naturopathy
F	65	Homemaker	Government-sponsored (Bhamashah Card)	AyurVAID
F	53	Homemaker	Government-sponsored (Bhamashah Card)	Cardiologist
F	27	Homemaker	Self-financed	Infertility issue
F	29	Homemaker	Self-financed	Oncologist
M	30	Government employee	Insurance	ENT
F	32	Private employee	Insurance	Gynecologist
F	38	Homemaker	Self-financed	MD
M	30	Private employee	Insurance	Orthopedic
M	75	Family business	Government-sponsored (Bhamashah Card)	Accidental case
F	32	Homemaker	Self-financed	Gynecologist

a) Familiarization with the raw data, achieved by rereading the transcripts and field notes.
b) Identification of the thematic framework, which entailed identifying recurring sub-themes.
c) Indexing the transcripts according to the sub-themes identified.
d) Charting and rearranging the data into the area of the thematic framework to which they related.
e) Mapping and interpreting the data; this involved the interpretation and categorization of the charts of data collected to create broader themes from the sub-themes.

Analysis began soon after the completion of the entire interview. By carrying out data collection and analysis concurrently, it was possible to employ an iterative approach to the investigation, such as findings that were used to shape the discussion in a subsequent interview. As the data interviews were progressed, data were analyzed and new themes added where necessary.

Themes

Six core themes were identified, each with their sub-themes which are described in the tables.

Table 8.3 provides a detailed description regarding attitudes toward domestic medical tourism.

Theme 1: Attitudes toward domestic medical tourism

This theme addresses (Table 8.3) how participants conceptualized medical tourism, what they understood about medical tourism and why they prefer domestic medical tourism.

TABLE 8.3

Domestic Medical Tourism

Initial Categories	Sub-Theme	Core Theme
Negligence by hospital staff (Shahpura Hospital)	Lack of facilities leads to move to Jaipur Hospital	Attitudes of patients toward Jaipur hospital
Lack of specialist doctor		
Lack of naturopathy and Ayurveda doctor in Shahpura town		
Better treatment and good facilities	Good experience in terms of accessing medical facilities in Jaipur Hospital	
Feel-good factor		
Availability of all generic medicines and shorter waiting time for diagnostic report		

Sub-theme 1a: Lack of facilities leads to move to Jaipur hospitals All respondents stated that a lack of specialist doctors and poor medical infrastructure and facilities near their homes are the prime causes to access treatment from Jaipur hospitals.

"I am a sixty-year-old heart patient, already suffer from a minor heart attack. In my area, there is no heart specialist from whom I can access treatment. For that reason I have to travel to Jaipur in the interval of every thirty days to get the treatment from Tongya Hospital Jaipur" (3M, 60 yrs).

Sub-theme 1b: Good experience in terms of hospital facilities Domestic medical tourism perceived as easy and patients have to suffer less while getting treatment from the Jaipur hospital.

Patient insight: "During my child's treatment from J.K. Loan hospital, doctors diagnose my son with great care and prescribe less medicine and that also generic medicine, where I have to spend less amount on medicines, and I am able to get a generic medicine in stores too" (1M, 7 yrs).

Table 8.4 provides a detailed explanation related to there being no language and cultural barrier.

Theme 2: No culture and language barrier

This theme explored the respondent's views on how the language directly influences domestic tourism, which is explained in Table 8.4.

Sub-theme 2a: No communication obstacle Participants identified the language issue as one that made them prefer Jaipur hospitals because people there were aware of their regional language and they can easily communicate with the doctors and other staff attending the

TABLE 8.4

Description of Different Themes

Initial Theme	Sub-Theme	Core Theme
People knew the regional language	No communication obstacles	No language or cultural barrier
Easily approachable		
Relatives and friends staying in Jaipur	Help in time of need	

hospitals. Apart from that, the respondents found the same eating habits (vegetarians) in Jaipur.

Patient insight: "I am a 75-year-old person. While getting treatment from Jaipur hospital I share my health issues with the doctors in my language and I find it more comfortable".

Sub-theme 2b: Help in time of need Several respondents found that the presence of relatives in Jaipur city helps them a great deal while getting treatment as such a relative could attend them at the hospital to assist them.

Patient insight: "When I met with an accident, those days my wife has to take care of me. In the hospital, there are no facilities to stay attendant, in those days my wife stay in my brother's place".

Table 8.5 provides a detailed explanation regarding the patient's accessibility.

Theme 3: Accessibility for patients

Sub-theme 3a: Accessibility: where patients can easily acquire and use the service

Effortless: Getting medical treatment in Jaipur perceived as easy and convenient, which acted as stimulant and encouragement for the Jaipur hospital to provide better medical treatment for the domestic patients.

Patient insight: "Jaipur is hardly 60 km away from my place easily, 24/7 transportation is available. So, for heart treatment, I prefer to visit Jaipur hospital".

Sub-theme 3b: Availability and convenience Jaipur hospitals are in high demand for domestic medical tourism. Most of the respondents found that for emergency treatment they preferred Jaipur hospitals, because the better medical facilities, availability of doctors and shorter waiting times make Jaipur hospitals more convenient.

Patient insight: "Once I met with a severe accident, without delay my son preferred Jaipur Fortis hospital. I received the best medical treatment without any delay" (M, 37)

Sub-theme 3c: Easy access to Ayurveda treatment Domestic medical tourism is in high demand because of easy access to Ayurveda or naturopathy treatment in Jaipur city, where the Aroham Ayurveda hospital provides good treatment with nominal charges where large numbers of patients can get better treatment with a fair price.

Patient insight: "I am very happy with the Aroham Ayurveda for best Ayurveda treatment and want to share my excellent experience with the visitors of the clinic. I was

TABLE 8.5

Accessibility for Patients

Initial Categories	Sub-Theme	Core Theme
Shorter distance to travel	Effortless	Accessibility
24/7 transport facilities		
Easy to commute		
Positive word of mouth regarding Jaipur Hospital	Availability and convenience	
Better administrative facilities		
Less expensive and accepts all financial support (insurance and Bhamashah)		
Naturopathy, speedy recovery	Easy access to AyurVAID treatment	
Ayurveda treating the root cause of disease		

suffering from fistula problems for the last three years but after the treatment in Aroham Ayurveda I have been recovered from this serious illness" (F, 37).

Table 8.6 gives a detailed explanation of drop-in expectations of government hospitals.

Theme 4: Drop-in patients' expectations in Jaipur government hospitals

Sub-themes 4a: Post-consultation This sub-theme addresses how participants' expectations have dropped toward the government hospitals. Participants share their pain points while seeking treatments from SMS and Janana Hospital.

Patient insight: "After my operations, the follow-up procedure is not at all good, I suffer lots after operations" (F, 63).

Sub-theme 4b: Biased treatment process This sub-theme addresses how participants suffer while getting treatment from SMS doctors. Government doctors mainly prefer their patients who first visit their clinic.

Patient insight: "In my queue one of my patients shared that his doctor prefers his patients who get the consultation from his own clinic" (F, 28),

Table 8.7 provides a detailed explanation of behavioral issues.

Theme 5: Behavioral issues

Sub-theme 5a: Lack of care and concern toward patients, especially old patients This sub-theme addresses how respondents suffer from several factors, like the harsh treatment of hospital employees and people who were always looking to make money.

Patient insight: "It was strange when I was discharged from the hospital and the compounder came and charged money from me" (M, 75).

Sub-theme 5b: Biased toward own people/Networking matters for getting treatment This sub-theme addresses how when participants wanted to get treatment from government hospitals, networking played a vital role in getting the treatment.

TABLE 8.6
Government Hospitals

Initial Categories	Sub-Theme	Core Theme
After treatment, follow-up is the big issue	Post-consultation	Drop-in patient expectations of government hospital in Jaipur
Government hospital, consultation duration is shorter		
Government doctor prefers their patients who visit their private clinic	Biased treatment policy	

TABLE 8.7
Behavioral Issues

Initial Categories	Sub-Theme	Core Theme
Government nurses' behavior toward the old patients is harsh	Lack of care and concern toward patients	Behavioral issues
Compounders' and cleaners' tendency is to make money		
In the government hospital, only networking works for accessing treatment	Biased toward own people	

Patient insight: "I have to call a ruling party member for seeking the hospital facilities in SMS".

Table 8.8 provides a detailed explanation of financial problems faced by patients.

Theme 6: Financial problems/No acceptance of Bhamashah Card

Sub-theme 6a: Less use of Bhamashah Card in private hospitals This sub-theme addresses how patients face problems paying high bills in private hospitals, because large sections of the private hospitals don't accept the Bhamashah Card.

Patient insight: "While seeking my treatment from one of the private nursing homes in Jaipur, I have to borrow money from lenders as they don't accept my Bhamashah card and the hospital bills are so high that I can't afford them" (F, 63).

8.8.2 Discussion of Results

Respondents have a practical view regarding the function and expectations of domestic medical tourism; from the study, it has been found that instead of allopathy, domestic medical tourists adopted the naturopathy and Ayurveda treatments. The study also found that good medical infrastructure, specialist doctors, the same language and culture and easy access to local resources are important elements that affect the decisions of domestic tourists from villages or from Tier 1/Tier 2 cities to travel to hospitals in Jaipur for better treatment. The main purpose of the present study is to discern the expectations of the domestic medical tourist who traveled from their hometown to these big cities to access better medical treatment. The study reported that the expectations of the patients toward government hospital have declined and the major determinants are: (a) lack of post-consultation by the doctors, (b) biased treatment policies (where government doctors prefer those patients who get a check-up from their clinic), and (c) lack of care and concern toward the patients especially older people. An additional study also found that "behavioral issues" are the major factors that affect the domestic medical tourists accessing treatment in government hospitals and the major factors are: (a) networking in the government hospitals playing a major role in accessing treatment in the hospital, (b) lack of care and concern toward the patients especially older patients, and (d) the last factor where patients suffer a great deal is the less usage of the "Bhamashah Card" or government-supported financial insurance largely not being accepted by the private hospitals.

According to Ehrbeck et al. (2008) medical travel is very relevant, and it has a direct impact on economic growth for the country, but for some reason, medical tourism studies didn't cover much about domestic medical tourism (Reddy et al., 2010). Hudson and Li (2012) first introduced the framework of domestic medical tourism and its impact on regional economies in the United States. Bowling et al. (2012) proposed and developed a questionnaire that captures the patients' expectations in the health domain. Adugnaw et al. examined a study on patient expectations in the context of the public health sector. This chapter concluded by discussing the expectations of the medical tourist who traveled from their city to another to able the best medical care.

TABLE 8.8

Explanations about Financial Problems

Initial Categories	Sub-Theme	Core Theme
Lack of acceptance of government insurance in private hospital	No use of government Bhamashah card	Financial problems
Huge cost structure in private hospital		

8.9 Conclusion

The present study concluded that there is a positive attitude toward domestic medical tourism; however, the present study uncovered several determinants (accessibility in the Jaipur hospital, good medical infrastructure, friendly staff behavior and patients are more aware of the Jaipur city). Also, it concluded that in recent times, the expectations of the domestic medical tourist toward government hospitals have declined, and it covered several factors causing this (lack of care and concern toward older patients, post-consultation patients were not followed up with properly and biased treatment processes were followed by doctors). Based on our findings, researchers recommended that every hospital strictly follow the post-consultation steps for patients who have traveled to a different city to access the best medical facilities. The present study is limited in terms of participants, and future research with a larger sample size can help in presenting more robust findings.

References

Available at: http://tourism.gov.in/wellness-medical-tourism

Available at: https://www.ibef.org/industry/healthcare-India.aspx

Available at: https://www.moneycontrol.com/news/business/indias-medical-tourism-market-expected-to-touch-9-billion-by-2020-report-4639931.html

Beladi, H., Chao, C. C., Ee, M. S., and Hollas, D. 2019. Does medical tourism promote economic growth? A cross-country analysis. *Journal of Travel Research*, *58*(1), 121–135.

Berhane, A., and Enquselassie, F. 2016. Patient expectations and their satisfaction in the context of public hospitals. *Patient Preference and Adherence*, *10*, 1919.

Bookman, M. and Bookman, K. 2007. *Medical Tourism in Developing Countries*. Springer.

Bowling, A., Rowe, G., Lambert, N., Waddington, M., Mahtani, K. R., Kenten, C., et al. 2012. The measurement of patients' expectations for health care: A review and psychometric testing of a measure of patients' expectations. *Health Technology Assessment*, *16*(30), 1–116.

Caballero-Danell, S., and Mugombo, C. 2007. Medical tourism and its entrepreneurial opportunities: A conceptual framework for entry into the industry. rapport nr.: Master thesis 2006:91 (2007).

Chakraborty, C., Gupta, B., and Ghosh, S. K. 2013. A review on telemedicine-based WBAN framework for patient monitoring. *International Journal of Telemedicine and e-Health*, *19*(8), 619–626.

Cohen, I. G. 2010. Medical tourism: The view from ten thousand feet. *Hastings Center Report*, *40*(2), 11–12.

Connell, J. 2006. Medical tourism: Sea, sun, sand and… surgery. *Tourism Management*, *27*(6), 1093–1100.

De Arellano, A. B. R. 2007. Patients without borders: The emergence of medical tourism. *International Journal of Health Services*, *37*(1), 193–198.

Ehrbeck, T., Guevara, C., and Mango, P. D. 2008. Mapping the market for medical travel. *The McKinsey Quarterly*, *11*.

Eissler, L. A., and Casken, J. 2013. Seeking health care through international medical tourism. *Journal of Nursing Scholarship*, *45*(2), 177–184.

Falkenberg, H. 2010. *How privatization and corporatization affect healthcare employees' work climate, work attitudes and ill-health: Implications of social status* (Doctoral dissertation, Department of Psychology, Stockholm University).

FICCI. 2016. *Medical Value Travel in India: Enhancing Value in MTV*. IMS Health, India. https://www.moneycontrol.com/news/business/indias-medical-tourism-market-expected-to-touch-9-billion-by-2020-report-4639931.html

Gaines, J., and Lee, C. V. 2019. Medical Tourism. In *Travel Medicine* (pp. 371–375). Elsevier.
Grail Research. 2009. The rise of medical tourism. Retrieved from: http://grailresearch.com/pdf/Content pods pdf/Rise of medical tourism summary
Gupta, A. S. 2008. Medical tourism in India: Winners and losers. *Indian Journal of Medical Ethics*, *5*(1), 4–5.
Han, J. S., Lee, T. J., and Ryu, K. 2018. The promotion of health tourism products for domestic tourists. *International Journal of Tourism Research*, *20*(2), 137–146.
Health Tourism: Destination of India. Retrieved from: https://www.ibef.org/download/Health-Tourism_091211.pdf (accessed June 02, 2019).
Hudson, S., and Li, X. 2012. Domestic medical tourism: A neglected dimension of medical tourism research. *Journal of Hospitality Marketing & Management*, *21*(3), 227–246.
Hyder, A. S., Rydback, M., Borg, E., and Osarenkhoe, A. 2019. Medical tourism in emerging markets: The role of trust, networks, and word-of-mouth. *Health Marketing Quarterly*, *36*(3), 203–219.
Javed, S. A., and Ilyas, F. 2018. Service quality and satisfaction in healthcare sector of Pakistan—the patients' expectations. *International Journal of Health Care Quality Assurance*, *31*(6), 489–501.
Kaur, M. 2014. Medical Tourism in India. *Indian Journal of Medical Research*, *3*(1), 64–66.
Kravitz, R. L., Cope, D. W., Bhrany, V., and Leake, B. 1994. Internal medicine patients' expectations for care during office visits. *Journal of General Internal Medicine*, *9*(2), 75–81.
Lateef, F. 2011. Patient expectations and the paradigm shift of care in emergency medicine. *Journal of Emergencies, Trauma, and Shock*, *4*(2), 163.
Medical Dialogues, https://medicaldialogues.in/10-4-lakh-registered-doctors-in-india-maximum-in-maharashtra-health-minister/ (accessed Aug.14, 2019).
Musa, G., Thirumoorthi, T., and Doshi, D. 2012. Travel behaviour among inbound medical tourists in Kuala Lumpur. *Current Issues in Tourism*, *15*(6), 525–543.
Oberoi, S., and Kansra, P. 2019. Factors influencing medical tourism in India: A critical review. *SAMVAD*, *17*, 9–16.
Reddy, S. G., York, V. K., and Brannon, L. A. 2010. Travel for treatment: Students' perspective on medical tourism. *International Journal of Tourism Research*, *12*(5), 510–522.
Ruiz-Moral, R., De Torres, L. Á. P., and Jaramillo-Martin, I. 2007. The effect of patients' met expectations on consultation outcomes. A study with family medicine residents. *Journal of General Internal Medicine*, *22*(1), 86–91.
Singh, L. 2014. An evaluation of medical tourism in India. *African Journal of Hospitality, Tourism and Leisure*, *3*(1), 1–11.
Singh, S., and Badaya, S. 2014. Health care in rural India: A lack between need and feed. *South Asian Journal of Cancer*, *3*(2), 143.
Turner, J. A., LeResche, L., Von Korff, M., and Ehrlich, K. 1998. Back pain in primary care: Patient characteristics, content of initial visit, and short-term outcomes. *Spine*, *23*(4), 463–469.
Ye, B. H., Yuen, P. P., Qiu, H. Z., and Zhang, V. H. (2008, July). Motivation of medical tourists: An exploratory case study of Hong Kong medical tourists. In *Asia Pacific Tourism Association (APTA) Annual Conference*, Bangkok, Thailand.
Yu, J., Lee, T. J., and Noh, H. 2011. Characteristics of a medical tourism industry: The case of South Korea. *Journal of Travel & Tourism Marketing*, *28*(8), 856–872.
Yu, K., Gong, R., Xu, F., Jiang, C., and Luo, Y. 2018. Key success factors in healthcare ecology integrated tourism development. *Ekoloji*, *27*(106), 351–355.

9

Study on Edge Computing Using Machine Learning Approaches in IoT Framework

Pramit Brata Chanda, Surojit Das, Sourav Banerjee and Chinmay Chakraborty

CONTENTS

9.1 Introduction

To illustrate the concept of IoT, the idea of edge or fog computing has been proposed [1–3]. Edge computing platforms support the mobility of devices and geographically distributed applications. According to this archetype, computing resources are made available at the edge of the network, close to (or even co-located with) end-devices. Placing computing resources near the devices generating the data reduces communication latency. Furthermore, network-intensive data can be processed and analyzed just one step away from end-devices, thereby reducing the bandwidth demands on network links to distant data centers. The ease of processing and storing data close to the devices generating them will enable new services [4–7]. Mobility and geographical distribution are indeed the key characteristics of IoT deployments that can particularly benefit from edge computing. A few representative applications include content delivery to vehicles, real-time analytics of data collected by mobile devices and environmental monitoring through geographically distributed wireless sensor networks. The concept of bringing content closer to end-users is not new. Content delivery/distribution networks [8] deploy resources that replicate content from a source location onto servers close to the end-users. Information-centric networking [9] is a similar approach for enhancing the internet infrastructure to explicitly support content-based routing and forwarding. However, the content delivery/distribution networks and information-centric networking paradigms are limited to non-interactive content [10]; for instance, IoT data can be cached at the edge of the network [11, 12].

The edge computing servers also provide computational capabilities and can host interactive applications that support user mobility. Furthermore, an edge computing platform can relieve privacy concerns as the data generated from IoT devices are stored and processed within nodes in the edge network. This means that data can be pre-processed to remove private information before being sent to the cloud [13]. Besides, the offloading computation to resources closer to the users (and data centers that are not far away) can help reduce the energy consumption at the end-devices [14].

From the year 2015 onwards, there are more than 7 billion mobile cellular subscriptions corresponding to a penetration rate of 97%, up from 738 million in 2000 according to the last ITU report [15]. This reflects the fact that the use of cell phones and tablets has exceeded that of computers and laptops. Besides, the rigorous and ubiquitous use of cell phones has been accompanied by an evolution in the mobile network architecture (2G/3G/4G/5G) and explosive growth of challenges for high bandwidth services (e.g. Video on Demand) due to the "big bang" of social networking and entertainment applications. Even with the evolution of both the nano-technological components and the storage capabilities of portal devices, they are suffering from low computing power and battery life, so they are not able to perform effectively, which calls for cloud computing involvement [16]. In the recent era, the cloud platform gives the solution of data centralization in the core mobile network which will offer rigorous bandwidth in addition to familiarizing high latency. Consequently, introducing some of the computing functions to the network edges (multi-access edge computing, MEC) has been newly proposed in the mobile communications system. According to the ETSI definition, MEC provides IT and cloud computing proficiencies within the Radio Access Network (RAN) in nearby proximity to mobile subscribers. Located at the base station or the Radio Network Controller, it also provides access to real-time radio and network information such as subscriber location or cell load that can be exploited by applications and services to offer context-related services [22]. The RAN edge offers real-time access to radio network information and location-awareness, as well as a service atmosphere characterized by proximity, ultra-low latency and high bandwidth. MEC will enable operators to open their Radio Access Network (RAN) edge to authorized third parties, allowing them to flexibly and rapidly deploy innovative applications and services. The internet has recently experienced an explosion in the number of connected devices adding a new networking dimension ("anything" connectivity) to the internet of the future. An estimate from Cisco indicates that 50 billion things will be connected to the internet by 2020 [17]. This will lead to an unexpected amount of generated data. Thus, the IoT "Big Data" will be about four Vs: Velocity, Variety, Volume and Value [18]. Hence, we will have many different models of generated data at different rates resulting in different volumes of data that will be stored, analyzed and used by IoT applications. Consequently, considering advanced data management technologies will be essential. Cisco recently introduced the concept of fog computing to enable applications on billions of connected devices in the IoT to run directly at the network edge [19, 22]. Data, computing, storage and application services to end-users are provided by both cloud and fog. Fog is characterized by its proximity to end-users and its dense analytics. It also supports densely distributed data collection points and provides advantages in entertainment, advertising, personal computing and other applications. Essentially, fog devices can be interconnected, and each of them linked to the cloud [20, 22]. Therefore, fog is an edge computing and micro-data center paradigm, suitable for IoTs. MEC is a special case of fog computing specific to mobile networks' geographical distribution, and its support for mobility, which provides low latency, location awareness, improved Quality of Service (QoS) and heterogeneity support. The fog computing paradigm is well-positioned for real-time big data analysis.

9.2 Review of IoT and Edge Computing

In this section, edge computing and internet-based ideas are reviewed. It also highlights the prospects for assimilating those approaches.

9.2.1 Internet of Things

The upcoming trend of computing may be superior to the computer-based approach of desktop applications [26, 27]. The IoT is assimilating into modern life swiftly, as a technology based on innovative ideas from past years. As an archetype, IoT visualizes several physical devices, such as vehicles, smartphones, sensors, actuators and other well-established devices. Succeeding several commercialized processes, such as smart shipping, smart city, smart grid and smart healthcare, human beings are non-functional IoT processes belonging with some home and work application. As a result, this technology might have some effects on users and become crucial to future life. This leads an important part of the business field. It conveys mostly vital things that will change the interest of the US in 2025 [26, 28]. Equally, the total of interrelated devices has increased in the population throughout the world. In 2012, the number of interrelated devices grew to nine billion [26, 27], and the predictable quantity of interrelated hardware may be up to 75 billion in 2020 [29]. IoT strategies will, therefore, be very much essential and important sources in areas like big data in the future. Here, three different communication models for IoT have been discussed.

9.2.1.1 Communication between Machines

This type of model signifies devices that may perform the task of data exchange with other devices without some central hardware assistance [26, 30]. They are capable of associating with others through several kinds of networks, and are not restricted only to the IP-based networks. In one example, Figure 9.1 displays a switch based on smart technology that communicates with a smart light over Bluetooth 4.0.

Hybrid communication protocols allow different devices to exchange information among device-to-device networks, which syndicate within the device with a specific communication protocol to accomplish the requirements of QoS. This protocol is frequently used in several applications such as smart home or electrical automation-based system, communicating between both via the packets transferring, and has a moderately lower rate which is necessary. The emblematic IoT devices are home appliances such as door locking, switches and smart lights, and small data packets are exchanged with these only. Using smart home devices as an example, protocol devices of Z-Wave are not able to communicate with Zigbee protocol devices [26, 31]. These issues regarding compatibility limit the choices and experiences of customers.

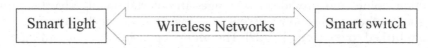

FIGURE 9.1
Machine-to-machine communications.

9.2.1.2 Communication within Machine and Cloud

In this type of model, request service of devices related to IoT from the service provider of the cloud, or saving data in storage of cloud [26, 30], because of boundaries of the ability of computation or capability of saving in the devices.

This methodology optimizes the existing communication mechanism and normally needs support from previous communications approaches, like several predictable types of connections, as shown in Figure 9.2. The various problems regarding the machine-to-machine model are solved in this type of model. But this type of model is reliant on the outdated network. The network resources and bandwidth affect the outcomes of the particular communication model. It is essential to elevate the network arrangement to fix the functioning of the machine-to-cloud communication model.

9.2.1.3 Machine-to-Gateway Communication

Here the model provides application-based middleware or proxy [30] services. Figure 9.3 shows the structure of the communications of machine-to-gateway. These schemes, as well as the algorithms, act an intermediary link within services based on IoT and cloud networks. This is supportive of the improvement of the flexibility issue of the IoT network and links a part of the computation job of the application layer. It expressively deduces the power depletion of IoT devices. A very popular and useful device i.e., a smartphone acts as the gateway in which various applications are running to communicate with different IoT devices and applications in the cloud environment. When a smart device is connected to the sensors which generate data, then a device with smart capabilities is required to encrypt the corresponding data by adding it to the service providers in the cloud framework.

9.2.2 IoT Components

Classically, types of components belonging in-network are associated with IoT: sensors, gateways or local networks of IoT, and the cloud service. The main functionality of these components is acting as data sources, networks for communication and processing information, consecutively.

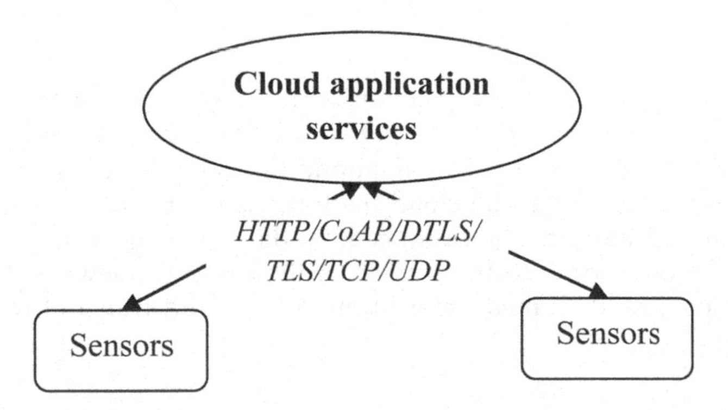

FIGURE 9.2
Machine-to-cloud communications.

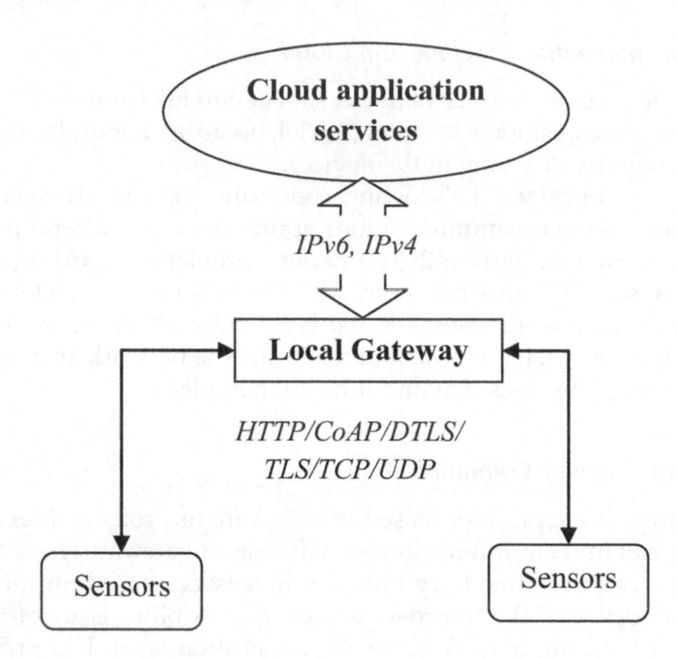

FIGURE 9.3
Machine-to-gateway communications.

9.2.2.1 Sensors/Devices

The sensor is a kind of device which can sense some physical environmental activity such as heat, motion, pressure and moisture. In the domain of IoT, a wide area can consist of millions of sensors. Those sensors are a crucial segment of IoT, and they do most of the data-measuring in the network. Those sensors may provide miscellaneous categories of information to help IoT which will be made aware of it. The users of devices can produce a majority of resource requirements and also the devices can serve as interfaces for human–computer interaction for creating user requests and accelerating them for IoT appliances. All of the sensors and end devices will be unified through the network so that they are able to exchange information with each other and deliver supplementary facilities.

9.2.2.2 IoT Gateways

The IoT gateways help to make a connection with the sensors via a network as well as with the cloud servers through the core network. When the end nodes of the network want the creation of resources for the IoT application, they direct the handling of data or storage tasks to the servers in the cloud platform. The sensors may be able to prepare a network to communicate the data produced. So they are needed to carry out data pre-processing before promoting it to the servers of the cloud framework. IoT gateways can accumulate and combine data measuring from devices and transmit it to servers in the cloud framework.

9.2.2.3 Cloud-Based Core Network

These servers accept data with requests from end-users through backhaul networks [26, 32, 33]. Another feature of cloud servers is that they have the capability of carrying out computations and data storage related to supporting IoT applications. Therefore, servers of the cloud platform can fulfill the needs for resources of several applications and send the outcomes back to the end-users after completing the data processing. In several applications with IoT, the end-users connect to cloud servers to accomplish the tasks of processing the IoT data.

9.2.3 Edge Computing

In the recent era, the number of mobile devices has rapidly increased. The latest 5G network technology is on the horizon [34, 36] and the edge may create an important way to address this matter. The major challenge to the fifth generation is Radio-Access Network (RAN) [36]. Edge computing for mobile provides information to RAN in a real-time framework. So providers might be able to give a better Quality-of-Experience (QoE) to users by using the RAN information in real-time. The reason is that the real-time RAN offers services with a context-aware model [26, 37]. It is specified that the edge computing approach permits nodes for responding to on-demand services, less bandwidth depletion and network latency. By this, the operators of networks can easily implement RAN in the edge for control by co-operators used by third-party owners, swiftly enhancing the deployment of the new application. The nodes which are participating in the computation are operating under the various co-operators, making it worthwhile to organize common schemes of security to ensure security at the same level.

9.3 Edge Computing Paradigm in a Cloud Environment

The edge computing archetype is represented in Figure 9.4 which provides the cloud computing platform support for data storage in the long term, and for statistical analysis. Edge computing as depicted in the cloud environment is explained below.

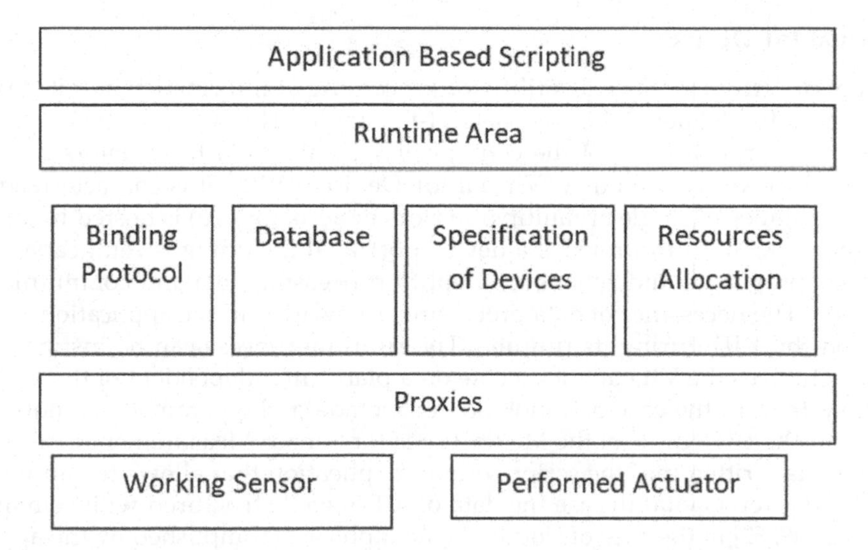

FIGURE 9.4
Functional components of a virtual IoT device.

9.3.1 Collection Proxy Technology

The sensors and actuators enable communications with many different technologies as well as protocols of communication. The collection proxies consist of software drivers and scripts for several technologies of communication (3G, Wi-Fi, BLE, etc.) and different protocols (HTTP, CoAP, etc.).

9.3.2 Data Validation

It is the primary stage of data processing of IoT where the sensor information is checked for some components [49]. This is obligatory, because sensors positioned in smart cities, agricultural fields and vehicles are susceptible to noise that can change the sensor data when it is transferred. Therefore, testing and the sensor data validation confirm that it is authentic. If it is found to be spoiled, then it is discarded. This procedure at the edge saves bandwidth and reduces the load on a cloud computing centralized scheme [49].

9.3.3 Annotation of Metadata

So, validated IoT data might be accurate if it is improved with supplementary data for the creation of metadata. For example, along with data about the temperatures of the agricultural field, the unit, timestamp, location and unique ID of sensors are crucial.

9.3.4 Security

Ecosystems of IoT may deploy several devices which cannot run critical encryption–decryption algorithms required for data security. The domain of edge computing is organized with payload encryption to AES-256 before creating communication to the area of cloud computing.

9.3.5 Virtual IoT Device

The concept of virtual sensors, its utility for processing of information and its taxonomy have been broadly deliberated in the state-of-the-art IoT [49, 50]. In Datta et al. [51], the work has given an extension of the concept of virtualization to actuators as required and proposed the conception of a "Virtual IoT Device" (VID). It is characterized as (i) a virtualized instance of single or multiple sensors or actuators; (ii) is hosted in an edge or cloud framework; and (iii) provides a device portrayal including several capabilities of those events, properties and actions to simplify processing data and communication to actuators [49]. The necessities of data processing are written in the application script that is loaded on the VID during its runtime. The runtime process can be instigated using Docker which gives the VID might execute on a platform independent of the underlying operating system. In the case of annotation of metadata, the parameters mentioned are used by us in the IETF draft of the Media Types for Sensor Measurement Lists (SenML). An approach is written into the script with an application that allows the annotation of metadata. This step is vital in case the data of IoT is well-structured with semantic web technologies [49, 52] in the case of cloud. The next phase accomplished by the application script is the processing of information whose logic will be influenced by the use of case scenarios.

9.3.6 Actuation

A very important utility of the architecture of edge-based computing is that it permits swift feedback through the actuation of different events. Once the local data processing is plentiful in a VID, if conditions are satisfied, it can elicit an actuation.

9.4 Edge Computing for Architecture

It is observed that the servers associated with edge computing are nearer to the end-user than cloud servers. Although the edge computing server's computation power is lesser than that of cloud servers, they deliver good QoS, with latency less than the number of users. Clearly, separate cloud and edge computing integrate edge computation with network [26]. The edge computation nodes communicate as edge or cloudlet servers. The edge computing structure may be divided into different aspects which are front-end, near-end and far-end, as shown in Figure 9.5. The dissimilarities in those expenses are defined here elaborately.

9.4.1 Front Structure

The devices (like sensors, actuators) are ordered for the edge-based computing block. The front-end domain can afford interaction better and provide better outcomes for end-users. Edge computing can provide real-time facilities for some applications as the computing ability given by a plethora of near-end components. However, for the lower capacity of sensors, most of the requirements are not sufficient to satisfy the front-end environment. Hence, in these cases, devices should send onward requirements for resources to the servers.

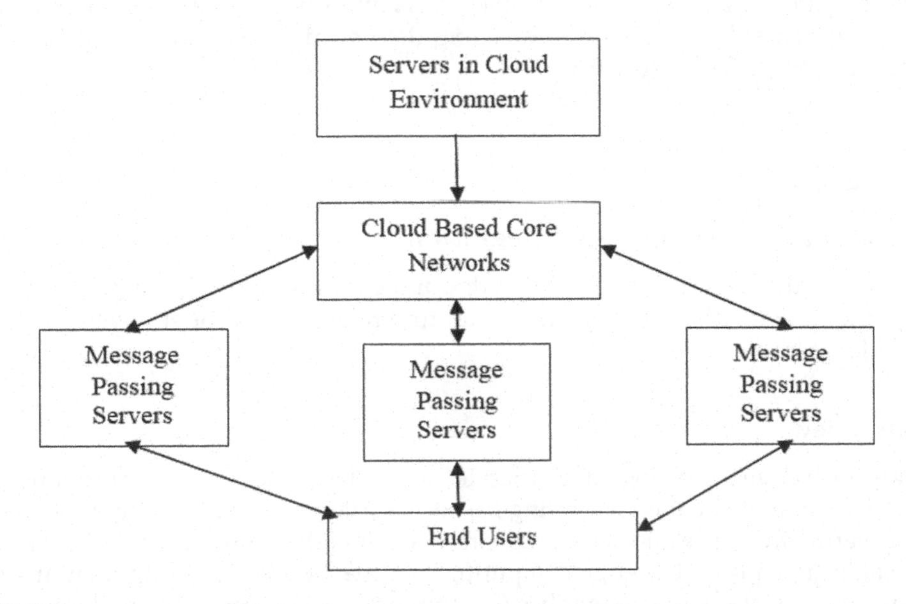

FIGURE 9.5
The basic edge computing architecture.

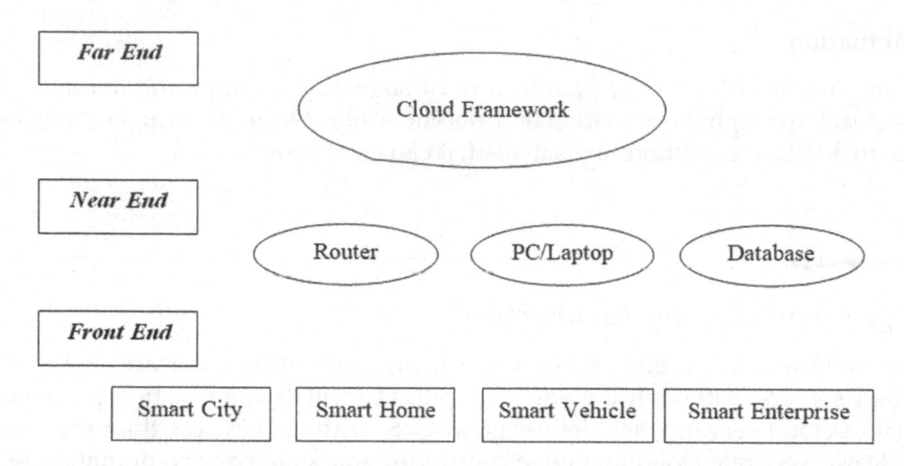

FIGURE 9.6
Architecture of edge-based computing networks.

9.4.2 Near Structure

The gateways are created through a near-end framework which supports most amounts of the traffic rows in networks. The servers, as they are edge-based, may also have copious requirements for resources like processing information in real time, caching data and computing loading [55–57]. In edge computing, the majority of data computation and also storage are changed to the near-end framework.

9.4.3 Far Structure

Cloud-based servers are supporting the end devices where the latency of transmission is substantial to the networks. However, the cloud servers located in far zone locations can offer more computing power storage capacity. As an example, cloud servers may deliver enormous comparable processing of data, big data mining, data management, machine learning, etc. [26, 32, 33] (Figure 9.6).

9.5 IoT and Edge Technology Integration

In this section, the characteristics of IoT, edge and cloud computing are discussed. It also provides the transmission, storage and computing-related tasks for enhancing the performance of IoT with edge framework.

9.5.1 Overview

The platform of edge technology may assist IoT to resolve some serious performance issues.

Figure 9.7 illustrates edge computing-based IoT's layered architecture. It is similar to edge computing in nature and sensors are the users for edge computing [35, 38, 44]. IoT can get assistance from both the edge computing and the cloud computing domains having the characteristics of several assemblies (i.e., the computation capacity and larger storage). Edge computing has additional benefits over cloud computing regarding IoT that consists

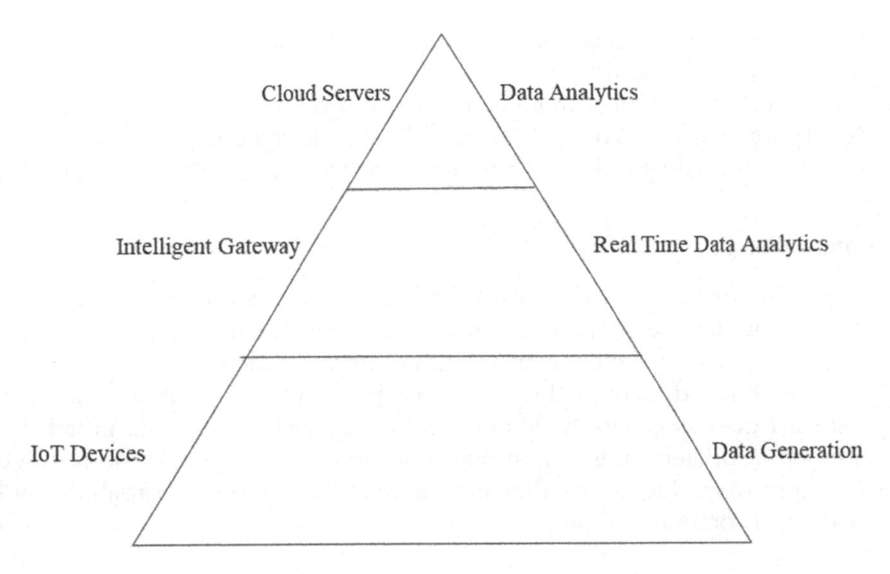

FIGURE 9.7
Edge-based IoT layered architecture.

of better capabilities of data storage and operation. IoT needs a faster response to compare to increased computational capacity and larger storage. Edge computing offers an acceptable computational capacity and sufficient storage space, as well as a swift response time for satisfying IoT application requirements.

9.5.2 IoT Performance Demands

Some specific factors regarding IoT performance demands issues are discussed below.

9.5.2.1 Transmission

Response time may be calculated for the addition of time of processing and transmission. On the whole, IoT devices produce a large quantity of data continuously and only limited computation requests [39]. Specific instances include communications of a vehicle and vehicle-to-infrastructure communications. Rather than a traditional cloud-based system, edge computing may offer plentiful computational nodes that follow distributed architecture; these are adjacent to end-users to support real-time data assembly and analytical services [26, 40]. The edge computation nodes also afford computational capacity suitable for handling lots of IoT devices. Hence, the IoT application requirements do not necessitate going through the delay in cloud services, as Amazon or Google Cloud without them may have the advantages of shorter time of transmission for edge-based computing [40].

9.5.2.2 Storage

IoT is the cradle of remarkable information that creates a significant part of the big data field, if not dealt with. Consequently, it requires adding immense storage and data to the edge framework. The advantage of adding to the storage of edge-based environments is, of course, the short uploading time. The drawback of this approach is the security issue with edge-based storage [26, 41]. Here, they are going in altered formats so it is very problematic to certify the information safety, privacy assessment, non-repudiation and cleanliness required for data [26, 42]. Furthermore, the edge nodes storage area is restricted and no other extensive and long-term storage connects with data centers in the cloud environment. In conclusion, when it is obligatory to add data, altered edge nodes will be engaged and synchronized for data gathering, enhancing the intricacy of data management.

9.5.2.3 Computation

As most of the IoT devices have narrow computation and resources of energy, it is too difficult to carry out on-site complex computational jobs. IoT devices can collect the data simply and pass them on for most computing nodes; in it, each original fact will be promoted for processing and analytical study. The capacity of computation of distinct nodes is inadequate. IoT devices generally do not necessitate much capacity and the IoT requirements can be appropriately satisfied, exclusively for services in real-time framework, by edge nodes. Moreover, edge nodes alleviate the reduction of power capability of devices over the loading of computation tasks.

9.6 Applications of IoT

There are several applications in the domain of IoT, and these are already used in areas such as: healthcare, travel and tourism, retail in business, hypermarkets, event management, the manufacturing domain, logistic systems, restaurant management systems and many others.

9.6.1 IoT-Based Industrial Applications

The working areas of IoT are gradually being enhanced today in the business domain with the integration of data processing in real-time environments, with properly utilized resources like data storage, payment online and QoS [74]. These are used to making industries with more profitable, effective real-time processing, development of competitive products, etc.

9.6.1.1 Smart Grids

For the past hundred years, there has been a huge rise in demand for electrical power. IoT has been used as an important technology for developing the electrical grid systems for smart devices. The traditional grid is generally based on analog meters for recording how many units of power are used per month for each household or industry operation. The evolution of autonomous and intelligent systems for smart grids allow comprehensive oversight on the distribution of energy which is effective for both producers and consumers [75]. These smart grid solutions are used to allow more accurate energy monitoring and supply them for controlling pricing effectively and also balancing the load for proper functioning of the smart grids. Also, energy consumption is performed by consumers in a real-time framework for other devices that might allow effective and reliable management of their energy. In the case of a smart framework, there are several requirements for the collection and integration of real-time data from each device within each household or industrial sector in IoT-based areas (Figure 9.8).

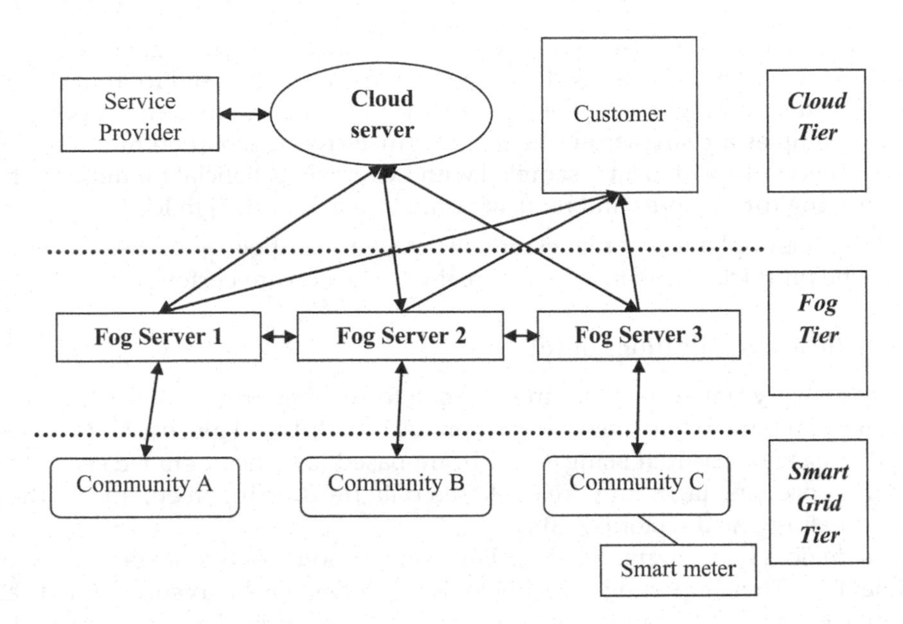

FIGURE 9.8
IoT-enabled smart grid in fog computing.

The architecture of grid systems consists of an advanced metering infrastructure (AMI) with area networks, data centers and substation centers with integrated systems. This architecture, AMI, uses communication in both directions and is performed with several devices with fog-based IoT nodes, which are a very secure, reliable and least cost-based service [21, 75]. The first tier is used for smart meters that are required for the collection of data regarding consumption of energy, as for inter- and intra-tier related communication. The second tier comprises the resource-rich network based on fog-based IoT mainly used for delivering computation-related services to this smart network. Lastly, the third-tier architecture is used for traditional cloud servers that are used for oversight and maintenance over the grid structure.

9.6.1.2 Manufacturing Process Monitoring

To improve throughputs and enhance the performance rates to optimize the resources, the architecture of the system is emphasized strongly.

Step 1: Gather the machine data from the environment to produce some information that streams some of the real-time data from several sensor-based networks and communication-based adapters that function on protocols like Simple Object Access Protocol (SOAP), Open Platform Communications Unified Architecture.

Step 2: The raw data streaming uses a private node associated with IoT-based machines which are crucial for monitoring the real-time natured data and provides time-sensitive control of devices to the production environment. It allows the system to work with a lower response time, improving the reliability and reducing the strain on the capacities of the network, as the data is being processed in a fog-based computation that is situated in the production environment in the IoT manufacturing framework.

Step 3: Here, several data samples are gathered for sending to higher performance data centers in the cloud-based framework which may be used for building models for maintaining predictive performance and optimizing the processes. As those samples are smaller in size that is transferred to cloud on minimal capacities of networks with data is sampled with extremely beneficial for industry-based improving throughputs and reducing unplanned items [75] in IoT.

Step 4: Next is applying this model for raw data, and tangible quantities are gathered into the production enhancement of real-time healthcare performance.

9.6.2 Healthcare Applications of IoT

The IoT holds very important roles in this zone for the betterment of services at a lower cost [76]. Several parameters, such as blood pressure (BP), blood glucose and body temperature can be easily measured using e-healthcare-based IoT. The upgraded sensors provide better data processing tasks for wireless-based data transferring in enhancing the uses of IoT in the health-related sector [77–81].

Medical devices have upgraded also, changing previous traditional devices to wireless related devices. This upgrading of technologies includes the emergence of medical-based IoT devices that are even connected to cellular phone networks. The health-related parameters are remotely recorded for back-end analysis of recorded data and providing the proper opinion of clinical experts. This is important for those patients falling into a critical situation, so experts can take faster decisions regarding diagnosis [76].

9.6.2.1 IoT Health-Related Service

This IoT-based system consists of three layers: information perception, network transmission and application service. The patient's health statistics can be continuously measured with the information perception layer [76]. Whatever data is collected is transferred through networks and gathered in cloud-based servers.

9.6.2.2 Glucose-Level Monitoring

In case of diabetes, patients require regular measurement of their glucose levels. A medical-based IoT system can continuously measure the glucose levels of a patient. The sensors which are wired so that they may be used by patients are required for tracking of several health parameters, and data items that are collected in IP-based networks. This network can track the glucose level of several patients who are associated with IoT-based networks within the healthcare area [76].

9.6.2.3 Blood Pressure Monitoring

The blood pressure of several patients can be measured with the sensor devices which are wired. It consists of network-based communication. Several IoT-based devices like Blipcare which can connect with a Wi-Fi network to record the BP level easily. It also consists of an LCD-related display [76].

9.7 Advantages of Edge Computing-Based IoT

In this segment, we discuss the various benefits of assimilating IoT and edge computing.

9.7.1 Transmission

The performance of network issues that can be measured by latency, bandwidth and loss of packets, within each other, upsets the transmission time. The faster data transmission time is one of the major advantages of edge computing, which can satisfy the QoS of time-sensitive requests, such as the "Live Video Analytics" project of Microsoft [26, 43].

9.7.2 Latency/Delay

The latency of an application is combined with two components: computing and transmission latency. The latency designates the time consumed on the processing of data that manages the capability of computation of the system. The devices frequently consist of implanted devices with a restricted computation capacity, while the servers of networks have a major capacity to afford quicker processing of data.

9.7.3 Bandwidth

It is not acceptable to transmit the corresponding data directly with cloud servers without data compression and processing. The huge amounts of data will consume vast network bandwidth and result in several disputes due to delay in transmission and loss of packets. Consequently, IoT gateways require executing pre-processing of information with aggregation before transmission to remote cloud servers. The tough task is mainly to regulate the amount of traffic to optimal processing of data, and tasks are aggregated to diminish the requirements of the bandwidth of the end-users, while protecting the numerous types of data.

9.7.4 Energy

The devices which are placed in the IoT network might also change the network's power resources – the capacity of the battery. Therefore, if the end device wishes to achieve the processing of data or bypassing it, it should sensibly have those factors in mind. It is imperative to exploit the total life span of end devices, particularly those with restricted battery capacity. If we want to achieve this goal, we have to arrange such a procedure as edge computing can combine an elastic task of the scheme of load data that may be power resources of the device. For example, Gu et al. [45] created the idea of fog computing-based cyber-physical systems in the medical domain hosting virtual applications in medical devices. With combined consideration of the association of communicating among base stations, allocating the subcarrier, an association of base stations for computing, deploying the virtual machine and distribution of task, a minimum complexity of programming algorithms of heuristics is anticipated to elucidate the combined-integer linear programming approach.

9.7.5 Overhead

In the case of transmission in the network, there will be overhead and payload of the header for every data packet. Edge computing has an open challenge for deduction of the overhead of the network. With the assistance of edge or cloudlet servers, packets can be amassed and pre-processing is done to moderate the needless overhead [26].

9.7.6 Storage

Classically, cloud computing-assisted storage is consolidated and created as a complicated, several-layer system, combined with servers and drives. These are erected in the most crucial areas and also the points of convergence in the topology of the network. Equally, some of the edge nodes are liable for demands of storage service, but in a difference from the cloud, an edge-based storage system is mainly distributed to the edges of the network structure. It correspondingly combines disk drives clusters, but also shares the requirements for storage capacity with several edge nodes [26]. To satisfy the requirements of QoS, storage based on edge computing can influence load balancing and also retrieval of faults techniques for the improvement of performance.

9.7.6.1 Storage Balancing

The IoT network devices typically have very restricted storage space. Different data is gathered or generated with devices and are passed on and saved in the server. Likewise, there are many devices producing huge amounts of data concurrently. If data is stored consecutively by devices in cloud-based storage, the outcome will be major network obstruction. For an example, the Microsoft "Live Video Analytics" project [26, 46] generates huge amounts of data, that requires sending storage less span period and requires incorporating in the process of an analytical approach in a given period.

9.7.6.2 Recovery Policy

The recovery policy is a vital constraint in edge domain storage, and dependability is crucial in storing and recovering perfect data representations. To increase the reliability, the system will crisscross the storage node's availability, data redundancy or redundancy of another node.

9.7.6.2.1 Availability

Typically, periodic pinging or a heartbeat is directed at systems to monitor for verification of system storage health and detecting the obtainability of nodes. Taking an example, a device might be unapproachable, based on edge storage nodes that might be damaged, or the hardware of the storage might provide an error, system mechanized repair method may eliminate or alter the disks' authorization, or the entire system might be closed for maintenance.

9.7.6.2.2 Data Replication

In IoT environs, the huge devices familiarize perpetual claims for storing data. The perfection of delicate data is authoritative, as health data, records regarding consumption of energy, for smart vehicles situations of speed or traffic, etc. Hence, the distributed storage systems must unavoidably implicate in IoT environs for succor to lever this huge mandate and cover data accuracy.

9.7.6.2.3 Computation

Each node consists of computation power lower than the availability of server nodes. Thus, computation tasks are required to allot edge nodes to fulfilling the edge demands. In general, a task scheduling approach is made to fulfill various types of objectives. In that area, several algorithms are considered for implementing task scheduling for edge computing.

1) **Computation Offloading**

   For obtaining better computation edge computing efficiency, the positions of the computation tasks must be adjusted.

A. *Local*

For IoT systems in modern areas, chips have become inexpensive and widely accepted. Therefore, the computing capability of devices has been highly improved. As a result, some of the computing tasks are carried out the machine-to-machine (M2M) network molded with a combination of IoT end-devices.

B. *Edge/Cloudlet*

Some computing resources are provided by the M2M network, but M2M is not adequate to meet the resource needs of all users. As a result, edge or cloudlet servers are required to provide the resources for IoT platform networks for the majority of users. To achieve this satisfactorily, the most serious issue is the edge/cloudlet server task scheduling. The balance required for scheduling servers based on the cloud is maintaining the optimality of servers with the stated limits on the assignment.

C. *Cloud*

The work shows that some processing of data or storage tasks necessitates more resources than M2M or Edge/Cloudlet can afford without considering all resources. In this regard, storage and computing power should be capable in the case of the traditional cloud. The servers consist of the largest in-network computational capacity, which means the achieved tasks on servers of the cloud environment have lower computation latency.

9.8 Edge Computing-Based IoT Challenges

The major edge computing-based IoT challenges are discussed here.

9.8.1 System Integration

Edge computing supports several kinds of IoT devices and altered service loads. Although it has so many benefits, it also has significant challenges. This type of computing integrates the various platforms, combining network topologies and servers. This may be problematic for program and resource management, with data for assorted applications running on variations of platforms in remote locations. The service providers in the cloud framework, such as Google and Amazon, have limits for allocating several applications and programs to run in appropriate areas and also hardware to make sure that the corresponding applications and programs are running appropriately [26]. Most of the users are unaware of how their applications are running or allocating their data and resources. That is the reimbursements of cloud computing as the services of cloud maintaining centralized architecture and handling easily. Here, developers face serious difficulties in making an application that can be implemented and executed in an edge platform. Some arrangements have been planned to improve the programmability of edge computing [26, 47] but these have not been considered for an IoT basis. Here, the primary phase is encountering edge nodes [48], which means before the process of discovery takes place, IoT devices are unaware of which types of platforms are used nearby. This is a big challenge for naming, allocation of resources, reliability management, etc. As for the huge amount of IoT devices producing and uploading data concurrently, naming data resources also becomes an immense challenge [26]. There are many outdated naming methods, like DNS and URI, and these satisfy cloud-based technology and upcoming networks.

9.8.2 Resource Management

The amalgamation of IoT-assisted edge technology requires proper understanding and managing of resources in an optimized way. IoT devices, frequently computing- and resource-scarce, will be greatly changed by congestion of network, applying power more to re-transmitting data in congested settings [26]. Edge computing, considered as a storage resource, can reduce latency issues and using resources in a decentralized manner will play a crucial role in attracting and sharing these assets. These resources can be led through a large variation, too long with itself computationally inexpensive. These connections must not be ignored. Indeed, the inspiring factors in these resources technologies coexist with several of those systems.

9.8.3 Security and Privacy

Both the moving goals that expanded in various zones and privacy are serious concerns that demand attentive reflection. From the point of view of edge-based IoT, those are, in fact, the most imperative issues [83–85]. Edge computing provides a focus on the complex intertwining of manifold and diverse technologies (systems, wireless, virtualization, etc.), and involves the espousal of an all-inclusive incorporated system for providing security that also manages every technology area in the entire system. Despite this lofty goal, the conclusion of computing will raise surprising issues regarding the security aspects [26]. The innate features of edge computing can alter sound edict types of security and privacy measurements are feasible and that could not be recognized [23–25].

9.9 Machine Learning Methodologies for Edge-Based Framework

Several learning-based approaches are indicated in various areas because of the uniqueness of solving problems with them. Those algorithms can solve machine-related construction in their way with knowledge [58]. Due to current technological advances, the new approaches are driven by making new algorithms with the use of big data technology to low computation costs [58]. ML and DL are based on advanced technology of several years used in huge applications [58, 59]. These are classified into three main categories: supervised, unsupervised and reinforcement learning. Supervised are based on prediction model mapping with learning [58, 59] and input parameter observation. In other cases, the methods use the relationships between parameters (features) and output.

9.9.1 Machine Learning (ML) Methods for IoT

Here, ML algorithms are studied i.e., decision trees (DT), support vector machines (SVM), Bayesian algorithms, association rule algorithms, k-means clustering and principal component analysis and their utilities in IoT [72, 73].

9.9.2 Decision Trees (DTs)

Each vertex uses a feature, and each edge uses a value that the sampled vertex is needed to classify. Those are classified as origin vertexes due to the values of the feature. These are the split optimal value of the training samples used to draw the tree vertex [58].

9.9.3 Support Vector Machines (SVMs)

SVMs are used for classification by creating a splitting hyperplane in the data attributes between two or more classes such that the distance between the hyperplane and the most adjacent sample points of each class is maximized [60]. SVMs are notable for their generalization capability and specifically suitable for datasets with a large number of feature attributes, but a small number of sample points [61, 62]. Theoretically, SVMs were established from statistical learning [59, 60]. The advantages of SVMs are their scalability and their capabilities of performing real-time intrusion detection and updating the training patterns dynamically. In another research direction, the results in Lerman et al. and in Heuser and Zohner [63, 64] showed that ML methods can break cryptographic devices and that SVMs are more effective in breaking cryptographic devices than the traditional method.

9.9.4 Bayesian Theorem-Based Algorithms

Bayes' theorem explains the probability of an incident based on previous information related to the incident [59]. For instance, DoS attack detection is associated with network traffic information. Therefore, compared with assessing network traffic without knowledge of previous network traffic, using Bayes' theorem can evaluate the probability of network traffic being an attack (related or not) by using previous traffic information. A common ML algorithm based on Bayes' theorem is the Naive Bayes (NB) classifier. The NB classifier is a commonly used supervised classifier known for its simplicity.

9.9.5 Random Forest (RF)

RFs have supervised learning algorithms. In an RF, several DTs are constructed and combined to acquire a precise and robust prediction model for improved overall results [66, 67]. Therefore, an RF consists of numerous trees that are constructed randomly and trained to vote for a class [65]. The most voted-for class is selected as the final classification output [59, 66]. RF uses DTs to construct subsets of rules for voting a class; thus, the classification output is the average of the results, and RF is robust against over-fitting.

9.9.6 Association Rule (AR) Algorithms

AR algorithms [54] have been used to identify an unknown variable by investigating the relationships among various variables in a training dataset. Subsequently, this model is used to predict the class of new samples [68]. AR algorithms identify frequent sets of variables [59], which are combinations of variables that frequently co-exist in attack examples. For example, in a previous study [69], the associations between TCP/IP variables and attack types were investigated using ARs, and the occurrence of various variables, such as service name, destination port, source port and source IP, were examined to predict the attack type. The AR algorithm reported in Mohammed et al. and Tajbakhsh [59, 70] exhibited favorable performance in intrusion detection. The researchers used fuzzy association rules in an intrusion detection model, which yielded a high detection rate and a low false-positive rate [59, 70]. AR methods are not commonly used in IoT environments; thus, further exploration is suggested to check whether an AR method can be optimized or combined with another technique to provide an effective solution to IoT security. The main drawbacks of AR algorithms in practice are as follows: the time complexity of AR algorithms is high, and association rules increase rapidly to an unmanageable quantity, particularly when the frequency among variables is decreased.

9.9.7 K-Means Clustering

K-means clustering is based on an unsupervised ML approach. This method aims to discover clusters in the data, and "k" refers to the number of clusters to be generated by the algorithm. The k-means algorithm applies iterative refinement to generate an ultimate result. The inputs of the algorithm are the number of clusters (k) and the dataset, which contains a set of features for each sample in the dataset. Firstly, the k centroids are estimated, and then each sample is assigned to its closest cluster centroid according to the squared Euclidean distance [82]. Secondly, after all the data samples are assigned to a specific cluster, the cluster centroids are recalculated by computing the mean of all samples assigned to that cluster.

9.9.8 Principal Component Analysis (PCA)

PCA is a feature-reduction technique that can be applied to transform a large set of variables into a reduced set that preserves most of the information represented in the large set. This technique converts some probably correlated features into a reduced number of uncorrelated features, which are called principal components [59, 71]. Therefore, the main working principle of PCA can be utilized for feature selection to realize a real-time intrusion detection for IoT systems; a previous work proposed a model that uses PCA for feature reduction and adopts softmax regression and a KNN algorithm as classifiers.

9.10 Conclusion

In this new technical approach, IoT-aided edge computing has become an emerging technology for cracking the problematic and complex challenges of dealing with millions of sensors/devices and the analogous resources that they require. Compared with the cloud computing approach, edge computing will drift data computation and storage to the "edge" of the network, near to the end-users. Thus, edge computing can reduce traffic in IoT. Furthermore, edge computing can reduce the transmission latency between the edge/cloudlet servers and the end-users, resulting in shorter response times for the real-time IoT applications compared with the traditional cloud services. Edge computing plays a vibrant role as a key enabler for the mobile and IoT-based domains that are receiving increasing interest in the research and commercial areas. Edge computing also supports applications that need intensive computational and real-time responses and it also plays a crucial part in serving applications with location-based mindfulness. Here, the investigation is based on edge computing architecture and several machine learning algorithms are used to scrutinize the edge performance for IoT-based application domains. Several health-related application areas have been studied thoroughly in this chapter and the relevant IoT-related applications were discussed briefly.

References

1. Gopika P., Mario D. F., and Tarik T. 2018. Edge computing for the internet of things: A case study. *IEEE Internet of Things Journal*, vol. 5, no. 2, 1275–1284.
2. Satyanarayanan M., Bahl P., Caceres R., and Davies N. 2009. The case for VM-based cloudlets in mobile computing. *IEEE Pervasive Computing*, vol. 8, no. 4, 14–23.
3. Bonomi F., Milito R., Natarajan P., and Zhu J. 2014. Fog computing: A platform for Internet of Things and analytics. In *Big Data and Internet of Things: A Roadmap for Smart Environments*. Springer, pp. 169–186, Switzerland.
4. Atat R., Liu L., Chen H., Wu J., Li H., and Yi Y. 2017. Enabling cyber-physical communication in 5g cellular networks: Challenges, spatial spectrum sensing, and cyber-security. *IET Cyber-Physical Systems: Theory & Applications*, vol. 2, no. 1, 49–54.
5. Wang K., Wang Y., Sun Y., Guo S., and Wu J. 2016. Green industrial internet of things architecture: An energy-efficient perspective. *IEEE Communications Magazine*, vol. 54, no. 12, 48–54.
6. Wu J., Guo S., Li J., and Zeng D. 2016. Big data meet green challenges: Big data toward green applications. *IEEE Systems Journal*, vol. 10, no. 3, 888–900.
7. Wu J. Guo S., Li J., and Zeng D. 2016. Big data meet green challenges: Greening big data. *IEEE Systems Journal*, vol. 10, no. 3, 873–887.
8. Frangoudis P., Yala L., Ksentini A., and Taleb T. 2016. An architecture for on-demand service deployment over a telco CDN. In *Proc. IEEE ICC '16, Kuala Lumpur*, Malaysia.
9. Ahlgren B., Dannewitz C., Imbrenda C., Kutscher D., and Ohlman B. 2012. A survey of information-centric networking. *IEEE Communications Magazine*, vol. 50, no. 7, 26–36.
10. Griffin D., Rio M., Simoens P., Smet P., Vandeputte F., Vermoesen L., Bursztynowski D., and Schamel F. 2014. Service oriented networking. In *EuCNC 2014*.
11. Li R., Harai H., and Asaeda H. 2015. An aggregatable name based routing for energy-efficient data sharing in big data era, *IEEE Access*, vol. 3, 955–966.
12. Li R., Asaeda H., and Li J. 2017. A distributed publisher driven secure data sharing scheme for information-centric IoT. *IEEE Internet of Things Journal*, vol. 4, no. 3, 791–803.
13. Satyanarayanan M., Simoens P., Xiao Y., Pillai P., Chen Z., Ha K., Hu W., and Amos B. 2015. Edge analytics in the Internet of Things. *IEEE Pervasive Computing*, vol. 14, no. 2, 24–31.
14. Ha K., Chen Z., Hu W., Richter W., Pillai P., and Satyanarayanan M. 2014. Towards wearable cognitive assistance. In *Proc. 12th Int. Conf. Mobile Systems, Applications, and Services, Bretton Woods*, N.h.
15. ITU, ICT Facts & Figures, The world in 2015 [Online]. Available at: http://www.itu.int/en/ITU-D/Statistics/Pages/facts/default.aspx (accessed: March 12, 2019).
16. Lewis G. A. 2014. Mobile computing at the edge (keynote), In *Proceedings of the 1st International Conference on Mobile Software Engineering and Systems*, pp. 69–70.
17. Evans D. 2011. The internet of things how the next evolution of the internet is changing everything. Available at: http://www.cisco.com/web/about/ac79/docs/innov/IoT_IBSG_0411 FINAL.pdf
18. Banerjee S., Chakraborty C., and Paul S. 2019. Programming paradigm and internet of things. In *CRC: A Handbook of Internet of Things & Big Data*, pp. 148–164. India: CRC Press.
19. Bonomi F., Milito R., Zhu J., and Addepalli S. 2012. Fog computing and its role in the internet of things. In MCC Workshop on Mobile Cloud Computing, pp. 13–15. New York, NY: United States: Association for Computing Machinery.
20. Stojmenovic I. 2015. Fog computing: A cloud to the ground support for smart things and machine-to-machine networks. In *Telecommunication Networks and Applications Conference (ATNAC), 2014 Australasian*, pp. 117–122.

21. Aazam M. and Eui-Nam H. 2015. Fog computing micro datacenter based dynamic resource estimation and pricing model for IoT. In *Advanced Information Networking and Applications (AINA), 2015* IEEE 29th *International* Conference on, pp. 687–694.
22. Ola S., Imad E., Ayman K., and Ali C. 2015. Edge computing enabling the internet of things. In IEEE 2nd World Forum on Internet of Things (WF-IoT), pp. 1–6.
23. Botta A., De D. W., Persico V., and Pescapé A. 2016. Integration of cloud computing and internet of things: A survey. *Future Generation Computer Systems*, vol. 56, 684–700.
24. Wen Z., Yang R., Garraghan P., Lin T., Xu J., and Rovatsos M. 2017. Fog orchestration for internet of things services. *IEEE Internet Computing*, vol. 21, no. 2, 16–24.
25. Wang L., Von L. G., Younge A., He X., Kunze M., Tao J., and Fu C., 2010. Cloud computing: A perspective study. *New Generation Computing*, vol. 28, no. 2, 137–146.
26. Yu W., Liang F., He X., Hatcher W. G., Lu C., Lin J., and Yang X. 2018. A Survey on the Edge Computing for the Internet of Things, *Special Section on Mobile Edge Computing*. IEEE Access, vol. 6, 6900–6919, doi: 10.1109/ACCESS.2017.2778504.
27. Gubbi J., Buyya R., Marusic S., and Palaniswami M. 2013. Internet of Things (IoT): A vision, architectural elements, and future directions. *Future Generation Computing Systems*, vol. 29, no. 7, 1645–1660.
28. Gupta A., Chakraborty C., Gupta B. 2019. Medical information processing using smartphone under IoT framework, Springer: energy conservation for IoT devices. *Studies in Systems, Decision and Control*, vol. 206, 283–308.
29. Rose K., Eldridge S., and Chapin L. 2015. The Internet of Things: An overview'. In *Proc. Internet Soc. (ISOC)*, pp. 1–53.
30. Wortmann F., and Flüchter K. 2015. Internet of things. *Business & Information Systems Engineering*, vol. 57, no. 3, 221–224.
31. Al-Fuqaha A., Guizani M., Mohammadi M., Aledhari M., and Ayyash M. 2015. Internet of Things: A survey on enabling technologies, protocols, and applications. *IEEE Communications Surveys and Tutorials*, vol. 17, no. 4, 2347–2376.
32. Yu W., Xu G., Chen Z., and Moulema P. 2013. A cloud computing based architecture for cyber security situation awareness. In *Proc. IEEE Conf. Commun. Netw. Secur. (CNS)*, pp. 488–492.
33. Chen Z., Xu G., Mahalingam V., Ge L., Nguyen J., Yu W., and Lu C. 2016. A cloud computing based network monitoring and threat detection system for critical infrastructures. *Big Data Research*, vol. 3, 10–23.
34. Yu W., Xu H., Zhang H., Griffith D., and Golmie N. 2016. Ultra-dense networks: Survey of state of the art and future directions. In *Proc. 25th Int. Conf. Comput. Commun. Netw. (ICCCN)*, pp. 1–10.
35. Agiwal M., Roy A., and Saxena N. 2016. Next-generation 5G wireless networks: A comprehensive survey. *IEEE Communications Surveys and Tutorials*, vol. 18, no. 3, 1617–1655.
36. Demestichas P., Georgakopoulos A., Karvounas D., Tsagkaris K., Stavroulaki V., Lu J., Xiong C., and Yao J. 2013. 5G on the horizon: Key challenges for the radio access network. *IEEE Vehicular Technology Magazine*, vol. 8, no. 3, 47–53.
37. Ahmed A., and Ahmed E. 2016. A survey on mobile edge computing. In *Proc. 10th Int. Conf. Intell. Syst. Control (ISCO)*, pp. 1–8.
38. Jararweh Y., Doulat A., AlQudah O., Ahmed E., Al-Ayyoub M., and Benkhelifa E. 2016. The future of mobile cloud computing: Integrating cloudlets and mobile edge computing In *Proc. 23rd Int. Conf. Telecom-mun. (ICT)*, pp. 1–5.
39. Bonomi F., Milito R., Natarajan P., and Zhu J. 2014. Fog computing: A platform for Internet of Things and analytics. Bessis N., Dobre C., (eds.), In *Big Data and Internet of Things: A Roadmap for Smart Environments (Studies in Computational Intelligence)*, vol. 546, pp. 169–186. Switzerland.
40. Georgakopoulos D., Jayaraman P. P., Fazia M., Villari M., and Ranjan R. 2016. Internet of Things and edge cloud computing roadmap for manufacturing. *IEEE Cloud Computing*, vol. 3, no. 4, 66–73.
41. Jiang H., Shen F., Chen S., Li K. C., and Jeong Y. S. 2015. A secure and scalable storage system for aggregate data in IoT. *Future Generation Computing Systems*, vol. 49, 133–141.

42. Hossain M. M., Fotouhi M., and Hasan R. 2015. Towards an analysis of security issues, challenges, and open problems in the Internet of Things. In *Proc. IEEE World Congr. Serv. (SERVICES)*, pp. 21–28.
43. Ananthanarayanan G., Bahl P., Bodík P., Chintalapudi K., Philipose M., Ravindranath L., and Sinha S. 2017. Real-time video analytics: The killer app for edge computing. *Computer*, vol. 50, no. 10, 58–67.
44. Niebles J. C., and Fei-F. L. 2007. A hierarchical model of shape and appearance for human action classification. In *Proc. IEEE Conf. Computer Vision Pattern Recognition (CVPR)*, pp. 1–8.
45. 45 Gu L., Zeng D., Guo S., Barnawi A., and Xiang Y. 2015. Cost efficient resource management in fog computing supported medical cyber physical system. *IEEE Transactions on Emerging. Topics Computation*, vol. 5, no. 1, 108–119.
46. Ananthanarayanan G., Bahl P, Bodík P, Chintalapudi K, Philipose M, Ravindranath L, and Sinha S. 2017. Real-time video analytics: The killer app for edge computing. *Computer*, vol. 50, no. 10, 58–67.
47. Raychaudhuri D., Nagaraja K., and Venkataramani A. 2012. MobilityFirst: A robust and trustworthy mobility-centric architecture for the future Internet. *ACM SIGMOBILE Mobile Computing Communication Review*, vol. 16, no. 3, 2–13.
48. Varghese B., Wang N., Barbhuiya S., Kilpatrick P., and Nikolopoulos D. S. 2016. Challenges and opportunities in edge computing. In *Proc. IEEE Int. Conf. Smart Cloud (SmartCloud)*, pp. 20–26.
49. Soumya K. D. and Christian B. 2017. An edge computing architecture integrating virtual IoT devices. In *IEEE* 6th Global Conference on Consumer Electronics, GCCE 2017.
50. Gupta A. and Mukherjee N. 2016. Rationale behind the virtual sensors and their applications. In *2016* International Conference on Advances in Computing, Communications, and Informatics (ICACCI), pp. 1608–1614.
51. Datta S. K., Bonnet C., and Haerri J. 2017. Extending data tweet IoT architecture for virtual IoT devices. In 10th IEEE International Conference on Internet of Things (iThings-2017), pp. 1–6.
52. Gyrard A., Serrano M., Jares J. B., Datta S. K., and Ali M. I. 2017. Sensor based linked open rules (s-for): An automated rule discovery approach for IoT applications and its use in smart cities. In 26th International Conference on World Wide Web Companion, WWW '17 *Companion, (Republic and Canton of Geneva, Switzerland)*, pp. 1153–1159.
53. Hype Cycle for Emerging Technologies. 2017. https://www.gartner.com/doc/3768572/hype-cycle-emergingtechnologies (accessed: March 12, 2019).
54. Mobile Edge Computing Market worth 838.6 Million USD by 2022, http://www.marketsandmarkets.com/PressReleases/mobile-edgecomputing.asp (accessed: March 12, 2019).
55. Edge Analytics Market worth 7.96 Billion USD by 2021, http://www.marketsandmarkets.com/PressReleases/edge-analytics.asp (accessed: March 12, 2019).
56. Khadija A., Micheal G., and Hamid H. 2016. Mobile cloud computing for computation offloading: Issues and challenges. *Applied Computing and Informatics.*, 14, no. 1, doi: 10.1016/j.aci.2016.11.002, 1–16.
57. CloneCloud: Elastic Execution between Mobile Device and Cloud, http://www.cis.upenn.edu/~mhnaik/papers/eurosys11.pdf (accessed: March 23, 2019).
58. Chakraborty C., Gupta B., Ghosh S. K., Das D., and Chakraborty C. 2016. Telemedicine supported chronic wound tissue prediction using different classification approach. *Journal of Medical Systems*, vol. 40(3), 1–12.
59. Mohammed A., Al G., Amr M., Abdulla A. A., Xiaojiang D., and Mohsen G. 2018. A Survey of Machine and Deep Learning Methods for Internet of Things (IoT) Security. In *Computer Science*, Cornell University, pp. 1–42.
60. Tong S., and Koller D. 2001. Support vector machine active learning with applications to text classification. *Journal of Machine Learning Research*, vol. 2, 45–66.
61. Vapnik V. 2013. *The Nature of Statistical Learning Theory*. Springer Science & Business Media.
62. Buczak A. L., and Guven E. 2015. A survey of data mining and machine learning methods for cyber security intrusion detection, *IEEE Communications Surveys & Tutorials*, vol. 18, no. 2, 1153–1176.

63. Lerman L., Bontempi G., and Markowitch O. 2015. A machine learning approach against a masked AES. *Journal of Cryptographic Engineering*, vol. 5, no. 2, 123–139.
64. Heuser A., and Zohner M. 2012. Intelligent machine homicide. In International Workshop on Constructive Side-Channel Analysis and Secure Design, Darmstadt, Germany, pp. 249–264.
65. Breiman L. 2001. Random forests. *Machine Learning*, vol. 45, no. 1, 5–32.
66. Cutler D. R., Edwards Jr T. C., Beard K. H., Cutler A., Hess K. T., Gibson J., and Lawler J. J. 2007. Random forests for classification in ecology. *Ecology*, vol. 88, no. 11, 2783–2792.
67. Meidan Y., Bohadana M., Shabtai A., Ochoa M., Tippenhauer N. O., Guarnizo J. D., and Elovici Y. 2017. Detection of unauthorized IoT devices using machine learning techniques. arXiv preprint arXiv:1709.04647.
68. Agrawal R., Imieliński T., and Swami A. 1993. Mining association rules between sets of items in large databases. ACM Sigmod Record. vol. 22, no. 2, 207–216.
69. Brahmi H., Brahmi I., and Yahia S. B. 2012. OMC-IDS: At the cross-roads of OLAP mining and intrusion detection. In Pacific-Asia Conference on Knowledge Discovery and Data Mining, pp. 13–24.
70. Tajbakhsh A., Rahmati M., and Mirzaei A. 2009. Intrusion detection using fuzzy association rules. *Applied Soft Computing*, vol. 9, no. 2, 462–469.
71. Wold S., Esbensen K., and Geladi P. 1987, Principal component analysis. *Chemometrics and Intelligent Laboratory Systems*, vol. 2, no. 1–3, 37–52.
72. Scherer D., Müller A., and Behnke S. 2010. Evaluation of pooling operations in convolutional architectures for object recognition. In International Conference on Artificial Neural Networks, pp. 92–101, Thessaloniki, Greece.
73. Ciresan D. C., Meier U., Masci J., Maria G. L., and Schmidhuber J. 2011. Flexible, high performance convolutional neural networks for image classification. In *IJCAI Proceedings-International Joint Conference on Artificial Intelligence*, vol. 22, no. 1, 1237.
74. Lee I., and Lee K. 2015. The Internet of things (IoT): Applications, investments and challenges for enterprises, *Business Horizons*, vol. 58, 431–440.
75. Chalapathi G. S. S., Vinay C., Aabhaas V., and Rajkumar B. 2019. Industrial Internet of Things (IIoT) Applications of Edge and Fog Computing: A Review and Future Directions, arXiv:1912.00595v1 [cs.NI].
76. Fayez H. A. 2018. The application of the internet of things in healthcare. *International Journal of Computers & Applications* (0975 – 8887), vol. 180, no.18, 19–23.
77. Suzuki T., Tanaka H., Minami S., Yamada H., and Miyata T. 2013. Wearable wireless vital monitoring technology for smart health care. In *Proceedings of the 7th International Symposium on Medical Information and Communication Technology*. Tokyo, Japan: IEEE.
78. Liu C., Yang C., Zhang X., and Chen J. 2015. External integrity verification for outsourced big data in cloud and IoT. A big picture. *Future Generation Computer Systems*, vol. 49, 58–67.
79. Ma Y., Rao J., Hu W., Meng X., Han X., Zhang Y., and Liu C. 2012. An efficient index for massive IoT data in cloud environment. In *21st International Conference on Information and Knowledge Management*. Maui, HI: ACM.
80. Yang L., Ge Y., Li W., Rao W., and Shen W. 2014. A home mobile healthcare system for wheelchair users. In 18th International Conference on Computer Supported Cooperative Work in Design. Hsinchu, Taiwan: IEEE.
81. Sivagami S., Revathy D., and Nithyabharathi L. 2016. Smart health care system implemented using IoT. *International Journal of Contemporary Research in Computer Science and Technology*, vol. 2, 641–646.
82. Chakraborty C. 2019. Computational approach for chronic wound tissue characterization. *Informatics in Medicine Unlocked*, vol. 17, 1–10.
83. Chanda P. B., Sarkar S. K., 2018. Detection and Classification of Breast Cancer in Mammographic Images Using Efficient Image Segmentation Technique, LNEE, volume 591, springer, CSPES.
84. O. B. Sezer, E. Dogdu, and A. M. Ozbayoglu 2018. ContextAware Computing, Learning, and Big Data in Internet of Things: A Survey, *IEEE Internet of Things Journal*, vol. 5, no. 1, 1–27.
85. J. Granjal, E. Monteiro, and J. S. Silva 2015. Security for the internet of things: a survey of existing protocols and open research issues, IEEE Communications Surveys & Tutorials, vol. 17, no. 3, 1294–1312.

Index

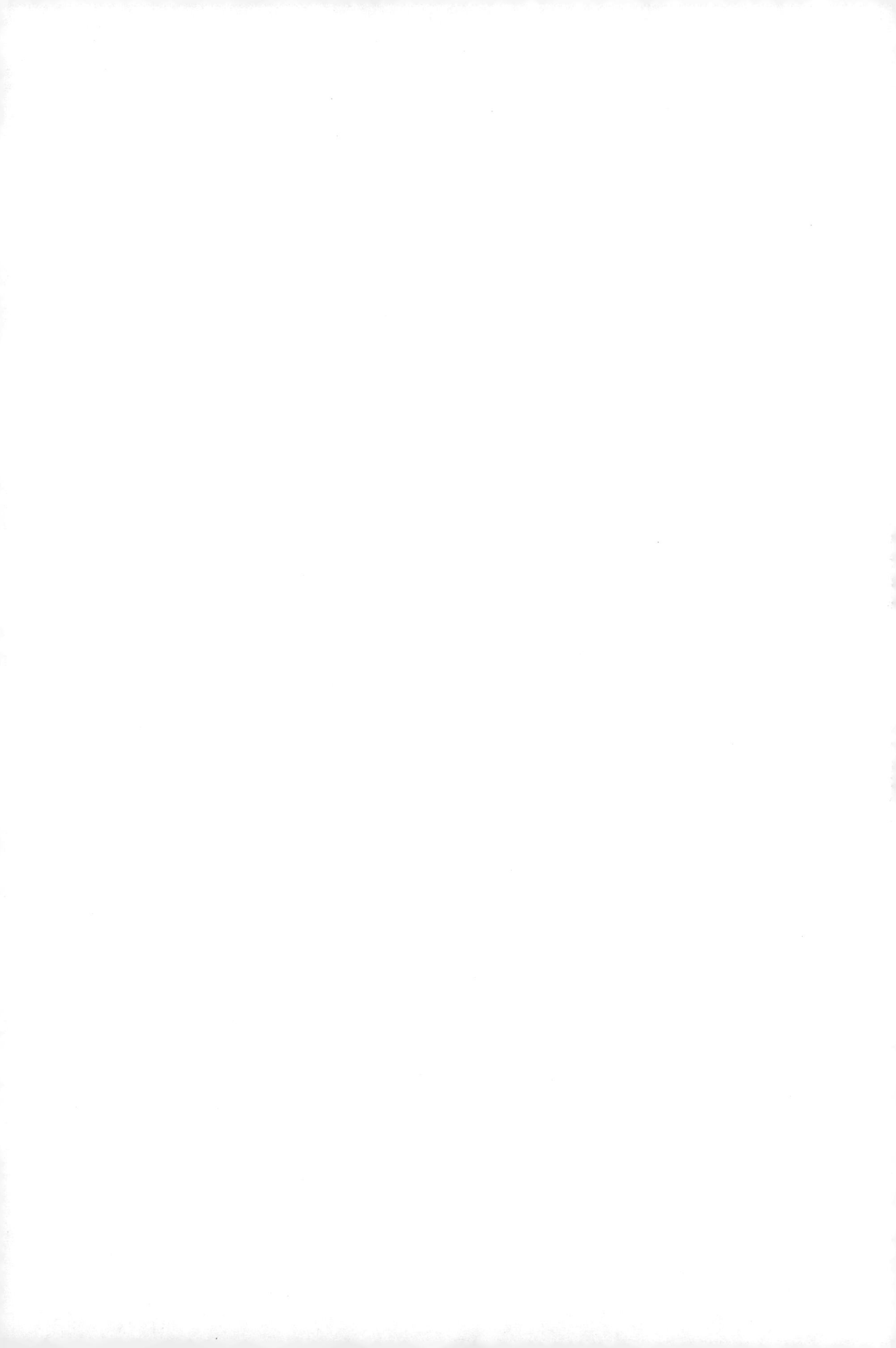